Vascular Ultrasound of the Neck

An Interpretive Atlas

Vascular Ultrasound of the Neck

An Interpretive Atlas

Antonio Alayón, M.D.

Attending Physician
Department of Neurology
Associated University Hospital Our Lady of Candelaria
Canary Health Service
Santa Cruxe, Tenerife
Canary Islands

William M. McKinney, M.D.

Emeritus Professor
Department of Neurology
Wake Forest University Baptist Medical Center
Winston Salem, North Carolina

LIPPINCOTT WILLIAMS & WILKINS
A **Wolters Kluwer** Company
Philadelphia • Baltimore • New York • London
Buenos Aires • Hong Kong • Sydney • Tokyo

Acquisitions Editor: Anne M. Sydor
Developmental Editor: Julia Seto
Production Editor: Donna Carty
Manufacturing Manager: Tim Reynolds
Cover Designer: Christine Jenny
Compositor: Lippincott Williams & Wilkins Desktop Division

530 Walnut Street
Philadelphia, PA 19106 USA
LWW.com

Printed in China

Library of Congress Cataloging-in-Publication Data

Alayón, Antonio.
Vascular ultrasound of the neck : an interpretive atlas / Antonio Alayón, William M. McKinney.
p. ; cm.
Includes bibliographical reference and index.
ISBN 0-7817-2534-8
1. Neck—Blood vessels—Ultrasonic imaging—Atlases. 2. Neck—Blood vessels—Diseases—Diagnosis—Atlases. I. McKinney, William M. II. Title.
[DNLM: 1. Neck—ultrasonography—Atlases. 2. Carotid Arteries—ultrasonography—Atlases. 3. Neck—blood supply—Atlases. WE 17 A324v 2000]
RC936 .A42 2000
616.1′307543—dc21

00-030208

---

10 9 8 7 6 5 4 3 2 1

CONTENTS

FOREWORD

This unique book puts the field of neurosonology into the best format for this new discipline—photographs which illustrate normal anatomy, lesions, and the course of abnormality over time.

Beginning with the normal configuration of the aortic arch with B-mode Doppler waveforms and flow velocities, the book proceeds step-by-step and illustration-by-illustration with extremely high quality pictures, no more than one to two paragraphs of explanation, and a precise reference for further elaboration of the topic. Each frame has been very carefully chosen from among the myriad which this vibrant, dynamic technology affords from the videotape on which it is customarily recorded. Though one always loses dynamics by using stills instead of footage, this is the loss that the printed page requires in order to gain "freeze frame" illustrations for careful analysis. The book continues through the carotid artery and intracerebral vasculature (which neurologists know backwards and forwards but cardiologists will find terra incognita) and a consideration of abnormal pulses due to alterations of the cardiac rhythm (though neurologists, as a group, are very insecure with this, it is elementary for cardiologists).

Because the quality is so vivid, one gets the impression that anyone could see the lesions but, as a former neurosonologist, I can attest to the fact that when the artery is pulsing, the lesions which are so graphically displayed may be difficult to visualize. The fact that these photographs are static adds dimension to their study especially for the beginner—in a manner similar to the methods used to display the segments of fast-moving animals or rapid action in athletic tournaments.

This book will take its place in the increasing libraries of neurosonology as an illustrated manual for use both by beginners and experts who desire to have an intimate knowledge of all aspects of the vascular events which may lead to cerebral circulatory disorders. These disorders begin at the heart and extend through the aorta, the cervical arteries, the intracranial vessels, and the draining veins.

James F. Toole, M.D.
President, World Federation of Neurology
Stroke Research Center
Wake Forest University Baptist Medical Center
Winston-Salem, North Carolina

PREFACE

The use of diagnostic ultrasound for the evaluation of extracranial vessels in the neck was initially introduced in 1954 by Holmes and Howry, who described a cross section of the neck visualized through use of a compound scanner. During the 1960s and early 1970s, Doppler techniques and scanning using primitive instrumentation were introduced. Real time gray scale, color-coded Doppler and pulsed Doppler, with the ability to rapidly record information using television systems, were introduced in the 1980s and 1990s. These developments offer a new dimension to the study of extracranial vasculature and blood flow. The recent development of on-line clinical techniques, training programs, and instrumentation makes this an exciting era.

This atlas is based on over 35 years of active research, clinical practice, and teaching. It is designed as a teaching and reference guide for interpretation including basic references to the appropriate literature. Active clinical cases with examples of numerous pathologies were used in its preparation. Pearls and pitfalls highlight certain principles. Questions provide a study guide to the text. They are carefully designed and will introduce new concepts to the reader.

Antonio Alayón, M.D.
William M. McKinney, M. D.

ACKNOWLEDGMENTS

The authors greatly appreciate the assistance of numerous students, fellows, residents, and colleagues. In particular, the authors wish to thank Anne Watterson, Larry Myers, Paul Tesh, Dana Meads, Linda Bell, Annemarie Johnson, Heather Kiger, Chan Lane, and Chris Sheppard. Without their continued support, interest, and expertise, this atlas could not have been prepared. Special credit is given to Drs. Charles Tegeler, Frederick Kremkau, Disya Ratanakorn, and William H. Williams. The authors also thank Anne M. Sydor, Julia Seto, and Donna Carty at Lippincott Williams & Wilkins.

This book was supported in part by the Dr. Manuel Morales Foundation and the Avant Neurosonolgy Fund.

CHAPTER 1

DUPLEX SCANNING OF THE CERVICAL VESSELS

Through use of high-frequency sound waves, diagnostic ultrasound provides a unique method for visualizing the cervical vessels. The identification of soft tissue anatomic structures and correlation with the patient's clinical symptoms offer both a challenge and an opportunity to the examiner. The primary goal of this atlas is to provide a comprehensive resource for neurosonography students, vascular technologists, radiologists, neurologists, cardiologists, vascular surgeons, and physicians practicing in this field.

Sonographic techniques, normal sonographic features, and diagnostic parameters, as well as major pathologic findings and references are presented in a manner that aids the examiner in gaining in-depth knowledge for proper interpretation. The references serve as a practical guide to the literature.

Interpretation of the ultrasound visualization of anatomy is dependent on the examiner's knowledge of anatomic relationships in the neck. The bifurcation is generally at the level of the superior margin of the thyroid cartilage, but it may be lower in the neck or under the mandible. Various views allow an understanding of the anatomy in the individual patient. The posterior view is used to visualize a high bifurcation. The carotid in a typical neck is 2 to 3 cm under the skin surface in all three positions: anteroposterior, lateral, and posterolateral. It is strongly suggested that the examiner take part in a cadaver dissection to best understand the three-dimensional anatomy.

A protocol for duplex scanning of the cervical vessels is presented in this chapter. A primary objective is to detect a critical stenosis. If the stenosis is more than 70% in size, the lesion is associated with an increased risk of cerebral infarction. This atlas also adds significant additional information regarding various normal and pathologic conditions. The protocol presented in this chapter may be modified to match the needs of specific patients or vascular laboratories to ensure that examinations of the cervical vessels are comprehensive and accurate.

The preliminary report for a duplex cerebrovascular examination used in our laboratory includes patient data, a short clinical history with emphasis on the present signs and symptoms, vascular risk factors, previous cerebrovascular surgery, and the findings of other diagnostic neuroimaging methods when appropriate (Fig. 1.1).

The examiner first palpates the arterial pulse over the carotid and brachial arteries. The palpation over the carotid artery must be done medial and below the angle of the mandible while rotating the patient's head to the side being examined in order to relax the sternocleidomastoid muscle. When palpating the carotid arteries, the examiner does not palpate both sides simultaneously;

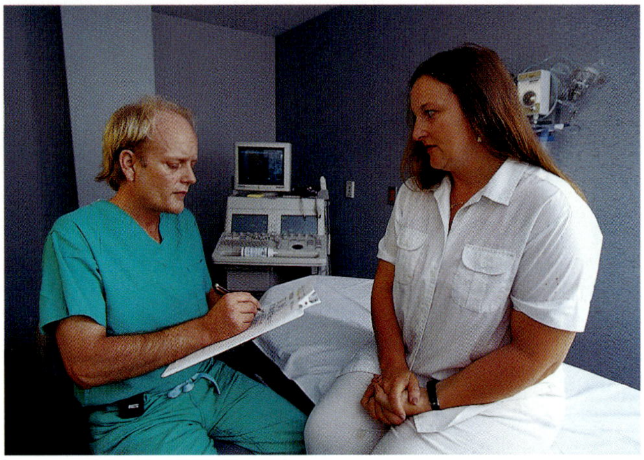

FIGURE 1.1. Clinical interview and preliminary report.

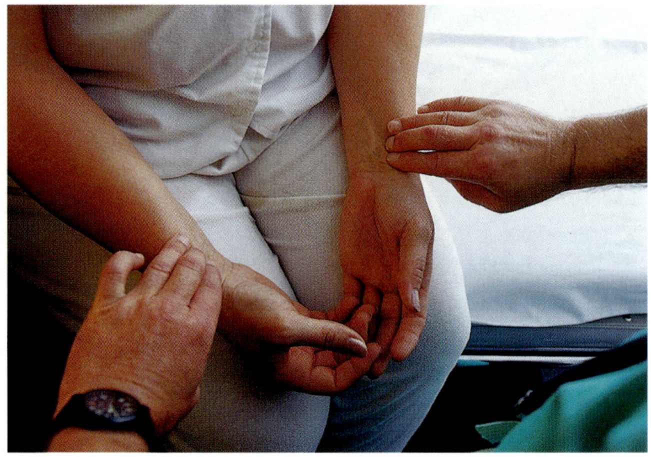

FIGURE 1.2. Obtaining the radial arterial pulses in the upper extremities.

excessive carotid sinus massage can cause slowing of the heart rate and a decrease in blood pressure, with resultant compromise of blood flow to the brain.

The arterial pulses in the upper extremities are examined to determine the sufficiency of the arterial circulation in the subclavian distribution. At least one pulse point of the radial artery is palpated in each upper extremity in the medial and ventral sides of the wrist, with the examiner using the distal pads of the second and third fingers (Fig. 1.2). Delay or unilateral absence of one pulse is a significant finding, suggesting subclavian obstruction.

Palpation of arterial pulses can indicate heart rate and rhythm, pulse contour, amplitude, symmetry, and sometimes obstructions to blood flow. The pulse rate is determined by counting the pulsations for 60 seconds or counting for 30 seconds and doubling the count. The resting pulse rate should range between 60 and 90 beats per minute. Bradycardia is defined as a pulse rate of less than 60 and tachycardia is defined as a pulse rate of more than 100. Next, the heart rhythm should should be determined. If it is irregular, it should be determined whether there is a consistent pattern. A patternless, unpredictable irregular rate may indicate heart disease or impairment of the conduction system. Lack of symmetry or strength between the left and right upper extremities suggests impaired circulation.

The examiner measures the blood pressure in both arms (Fig. 1.3). Indirect measurements of blood pressure are made with a stethoscope and a properly calibrated aneroid sphygmomanometer. The sphygmomanometer is composed of a cuff with an inflatable bladder, a pressure manometer, and a rubber hand bulb with a pressure control valve. The bladder width should not exceed two thirds of the length of the upper or lower arms and should ideally cover three fourths of the circumference of the extremity. Slow or repeated inflation of the cuff causes venous congestion and results in inaccurate readings. If repeated measurements are needed, a pause of at least 15 seconds between readings or elevating the arm for 1 to 2 minutes is suggested. The American Heart Association recommends recordings as follows: systolic and diastolic pressure. Two consecutive sounds indicate the systolic pressure. When the sounds disappear, it should correspond to the diastolic pressure. The blood pressure must be

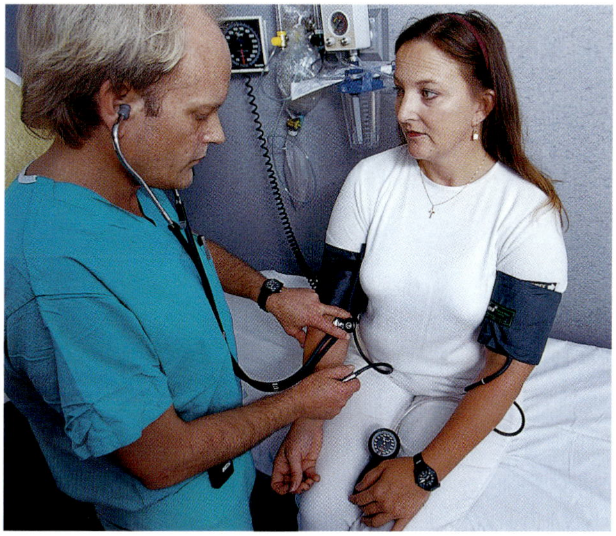

FIGURE 1.3. Blood pressure readings are obtained in both arms.

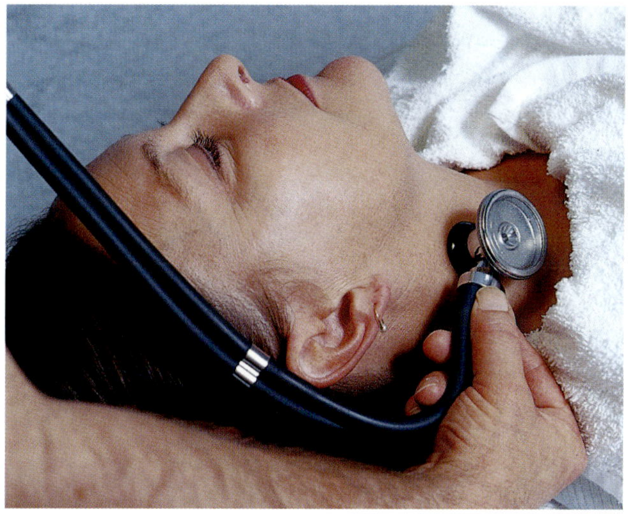

FIGURE 1.4. Systematic vascular auscultation of the carotid bifurcation.

read in both arms and may vary by as much as 10 mm Hg. The standard that is used for adults was set for patients in the seated position.

Auscultation of the skull and neck are routinely performed. The bell of the stethoscope is more effective than the diaphragm in transmitting the low-pitched sound produced by the turbulence of blood flow in the artery. Having the patient hold his or her breath for a few heartbeats helps the examiner hear more clearly. Sites to auscultate for a bruit are the common carotid bifurcation, the internal carotid artery, the supraclavicular fossa at the medial end of the clavicle, over the orbit, and below the occiput (Figs. 1.4 through 1.7). Mild obstruction produces a short, localized bruit. Greater obstruction lengthens the duration and increases the pitch. Complete obstruction eliminates the bruit.

The duplex examination of the cervical vessels should be performed with appropriate instrumentation, including high-frequency transducers and a

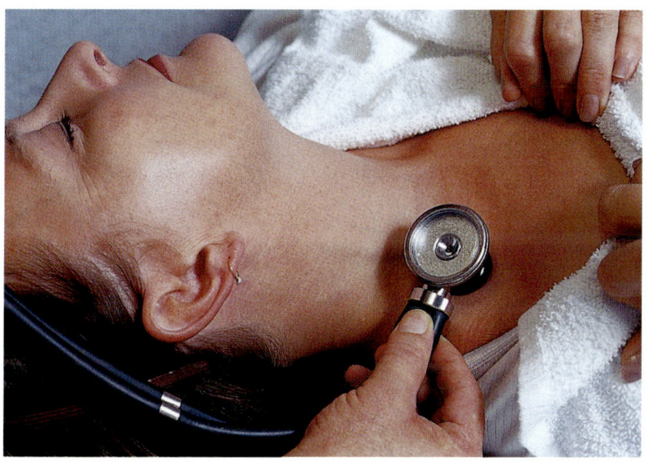

FIGURE 1.5. Systematic vascular auscultation of the supra-clavicular area.

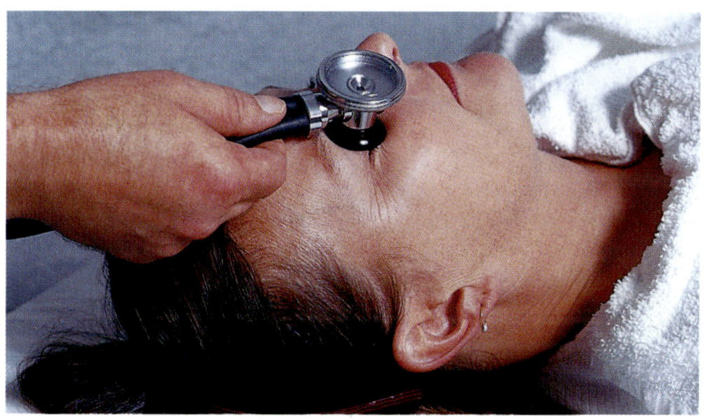

FIGURE 1.6. Systematic vascular auscultation of the orbit.

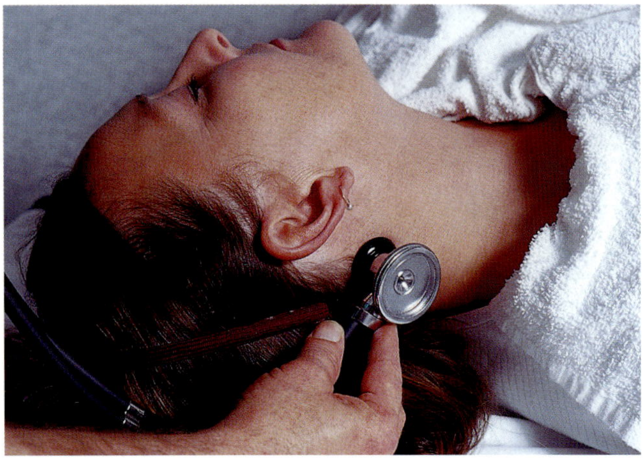

FIGURE 1.7. Systemic vascular auscultation of the occiput.

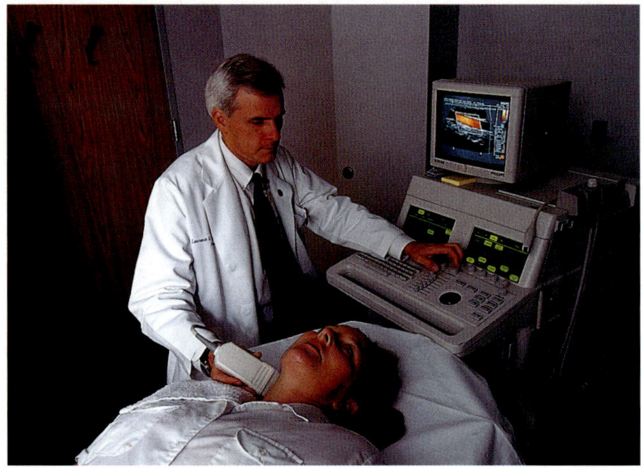

FIGURE 1.8. Proper patient positioning for ultrasound examination of the cervical vessels.

pulsed directional Doppler instrument with velocity measurement capabilities, variable sample volume, and online frequency spectrum analysis. Color duplex facilitates cervical vessel assessment and the volume flow rate should be measured in cases of stenotic flow.

The cervical vessels are examined with the patient in a supine position with the examiner seated at the patient's head (Fig. 1.8). Neck exposure is facilitated by having the patient drop the ipsilateral shoulder, then tilting and rotating the patient's head away from the side being examined. The carotid system is imaged from four longitudinal transducer positions: anteroposterior, lateral, posterolateral, and transverse (Figs. 1.9 through 1.12).

The duplex vertebral examination is performed in conjunction with the carotid examination. The patient is positioned in the same manner as for a carotid examination (Fig. 1.13). The image plane is then changed laterally until shadows (cast from the transverse processes of the vertebra) are located. The image plane is then changed until one or more segments of the vertebral arteries are seen between the transverse processes.

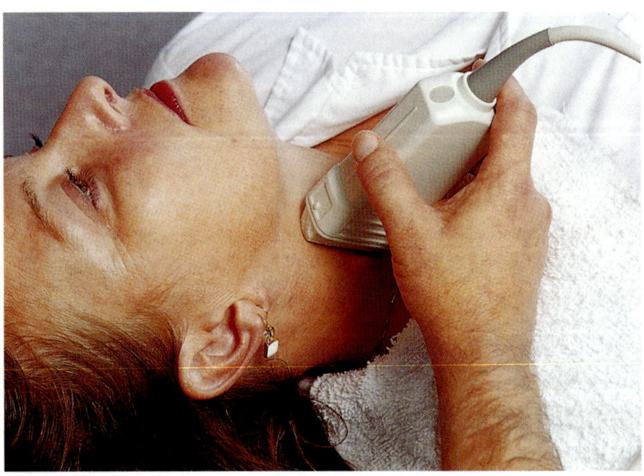

FIGURE 1.9. Imaging the carotid system: anteroposterior position.

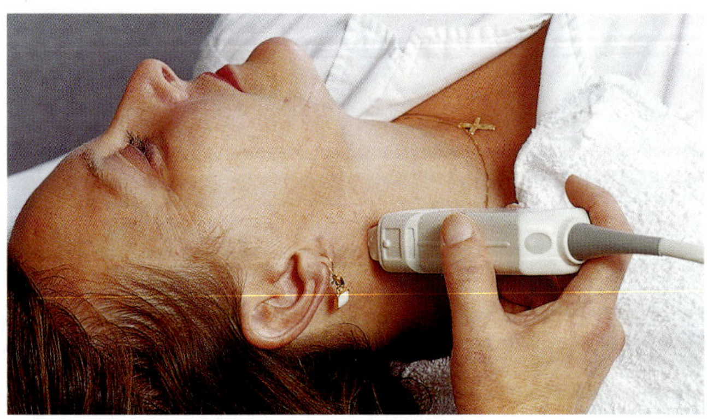

FIGURE 1.10. Imaging the carotid system: lateral position.

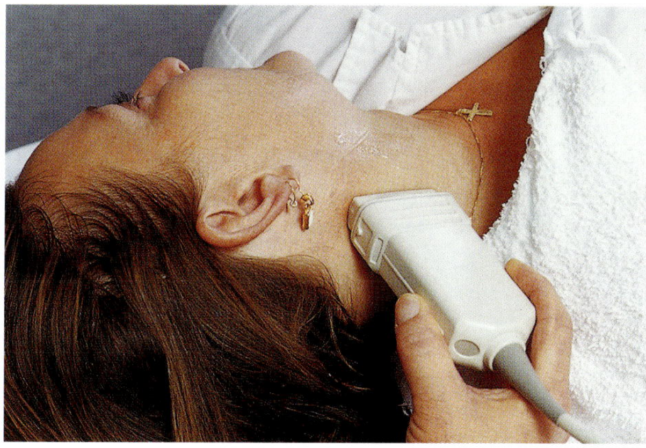

FIGURE 1.11. Imaging the carotid system: posterolateral position.

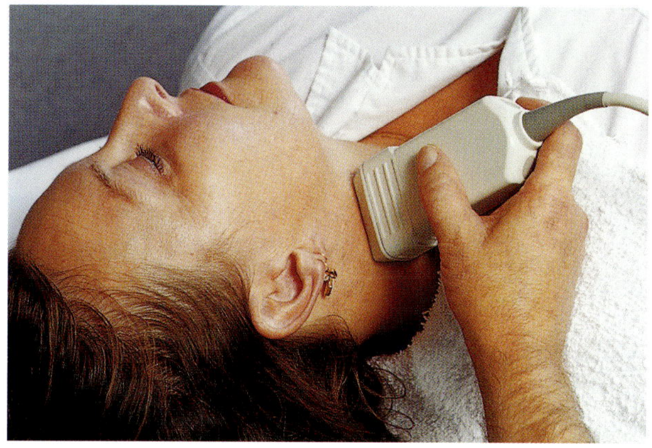

FIGURE 1.12. Imaging the carotid system: transverse position.

A record of the entire examination is made on videotape and includes verbal comments by the examiner regarding the locations and any abnormal findings. Clinical information, spectrum analysis, flow measurements, plaque location, plaque size, and severity of the cervical vessel lesions are recorded by the examiner in a preliminary report.

An emergency event may occur during the examination. Personnel should be well trained in the use of the following equipment (Fig. 1.14): choice of appropriate endotracheal tube size and lip-tip length, laryngoscope; suction catheter; stylet; oral airway; bag-valve mask; oxygen mask; vascular access catheter/butterfly; nasogastric tube; blood pressure cuff; defibrillator.

The examination is dependent upon the skill and experience of the examiner, a carefully followed routine, and a knowledge of underlying normal and pathophysiologic conditions. This atlas provides a background of basic information to complement this knowledge.

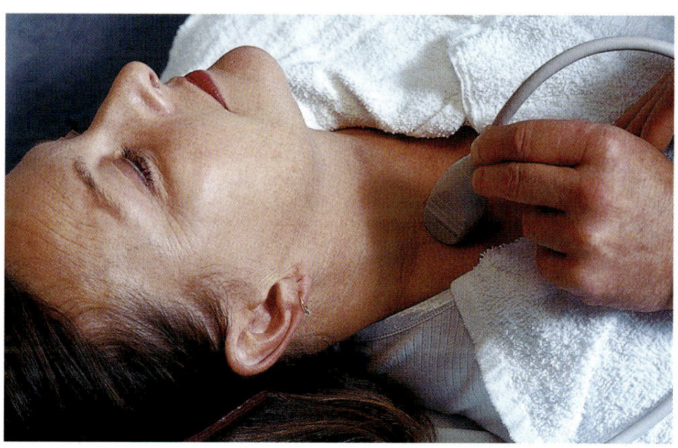

FIGURE 1.13. Imaging the duplex vertebral system position.

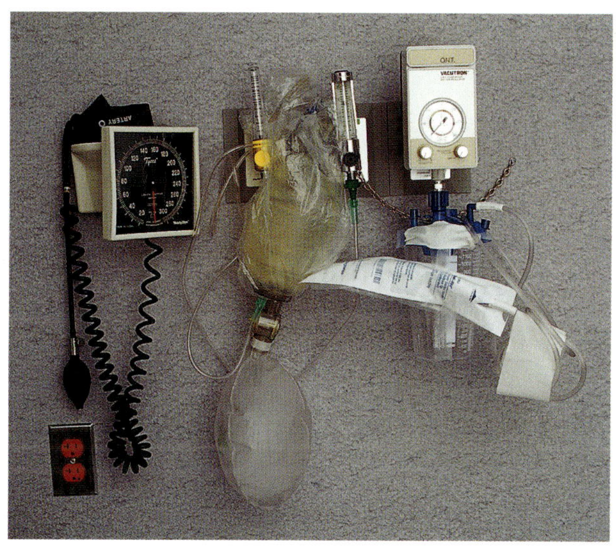

FIGURE 1.14. Emergency equipment that should be available during the examination.

SUGGESTED READINGS

Seidel HM, Ball JW, Dains JE, et al. *Mosby's guide to the physical examination,* 4th ed. Chicago: Mosby, 1999.

Tegeler CH, Babikian VL, Gomez CR. *Neurosonology.* Chicago: Mosby–Year Book, 1996.

Zwiebel WJ. *Introduction to vascular ultrasonography,* 3rd ed. Philadelphia: WB Saunders, 1992.

CHAPTER 2

NORMAL ANATOMY OF THE AORTIC ARCH AND CAROTID SYSTEM

Six brachial arches and clefts form during the early stages of embryonic development. Some of them remain to form the brachiocephalic artery. In the normal situation, which occurs with an overall frequency of about 70%, the right carotid artery arises from the innominate artery after its take-off from the arch of the aorta. The left common carotid artery arises as a separate trunk from the arch of the aorta and the left subclavian artery arises just distal to the former (Figs. 2.1 and 2.2).

The bifurcation of the carotid arteries into the internal and external carotid arteries is often related to the larynx. It is more reliable, however, to relate to the bifurcation to the vertebral column to avoid different heights of division according to the age-dependent height of the larynx. Typically, the bifurcation occurs at the level of the fourth cervical vertebra and differences of up to the height of one cervical vertebra have been described between the right and the left side. Usually the bifurcation of the common carotid artery occurs at the level of C3 on the right side in 30% of cases and at the level of C4 on the left side in 35% of cases.

At the bifurcation, the internal carotid artery usually courses lateral and posterior to the external carotid artery. The first branch of the internal carotid artery is the ophthalmic artery, which arises from the carotid siphon. The first branch of the external carotid artery, just above the bifurcation, is the superior thyroid artery in 50% of cases.

This chapter describes the normal anatomy of the aortic arch and carotid system by B-mode imaging in anteroposterior, lateral, posterolateral, and transverse views. The relationships are illustrated.

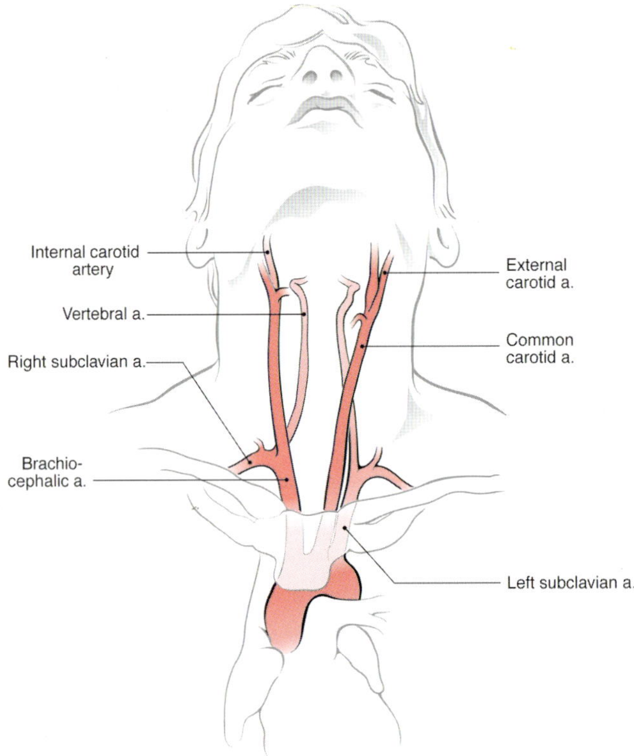

FIGURE 2.1. Major cervical arterial vessels.

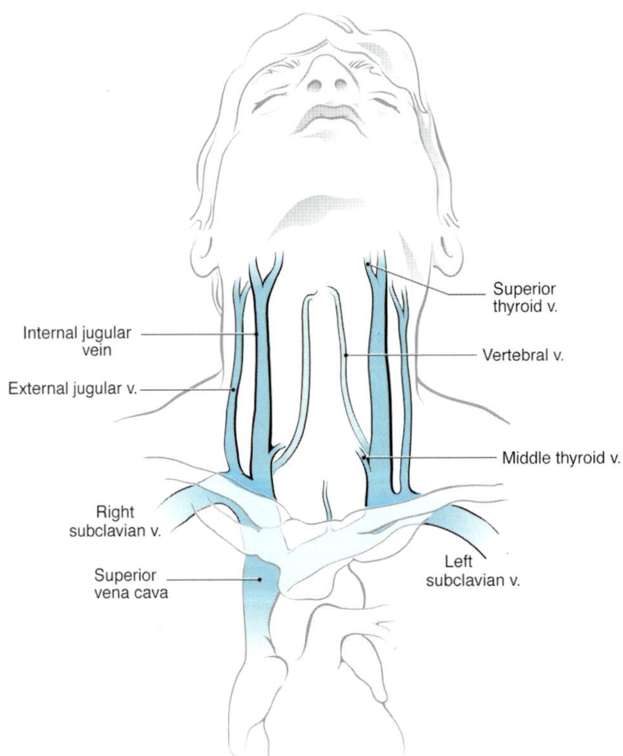

FIGURE 2.2. Major cervical venous vessels.

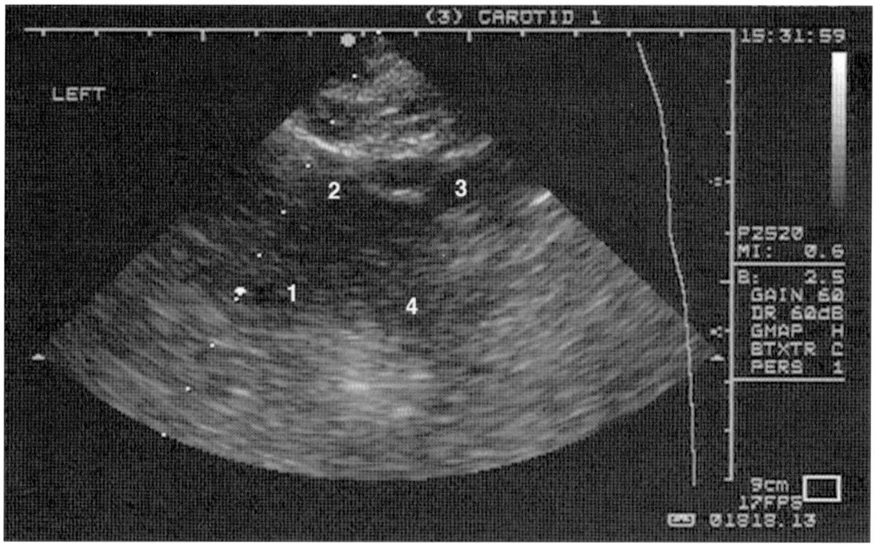

FIGURE 2.3. Aortic arch. Suprasternal approach. Longitudinal. Gray scale. *1,* Ascending aorta; *2,* innominate artery; *3,* origin of the left common carotid artery versus subclavian artery; *4,* descending aorta.

Diagnosis: Ascending aorta, descending aorta, and aortic arch. Normal anatomy. The aortic arch is the continuation of the ascending aorta. The arch first ascends diagonally back and to the left over the anterior surface of the trachea, then back across its left side, and finally descending left of the fourth thoracic vertebral body, continuing as the descending aorta.

The principal anatomic relations are as follows: anteriorly and to the left—left mediastinal pleura, left phrenic nerve, left lower cervical vagal cardiac branch, left superior cervical sympathetic cardiac branch, and left vagus; posterior to the right—trachea, deep cardiac plexus, left recurrent laryngeal nerve, esophagus, thoracic duct, and vertebral column; above—the brachiocephalic artery, left common carotid, and left subclavian artery; below—pulmonary artery bifurcation (1).

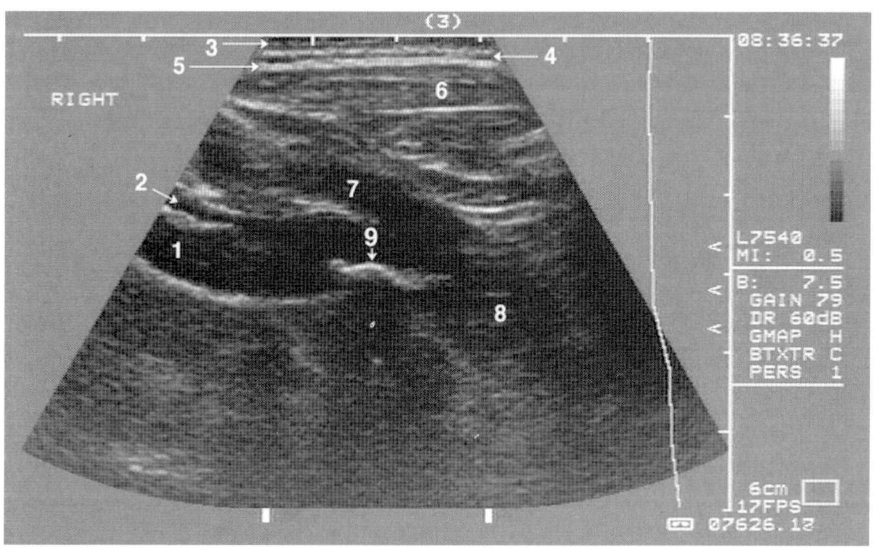

FIGURE 2.4. Brachiocephalic artery. Anteroposterior view. Supraclavicular approach. Gray scale. *1,* Right subclavian artery; *2,* right vertebral artery; *3,* skin and superficial cervical fascia; *4,* platysma; *5,* deep cervical fascia; *6,* sternocleidomastoid muscle; *7,* right common carotid artery; *8,* innominate artery; *9,* calcific plaque with acoustic shadowing at the origin of the right subclavian artery.

Diagnosis: Brachiocephalic artery. Normal anatomy. The brachiocephalic artery is the largest branch of the aortic arch, arising from the convexity posterior to the center of the manubrium. At the level of the right sternoclavicular joint it divides into the right common carotid and subclavian arteries. Anteriorly are the sternohyoid and sternothyroid muscles (1).

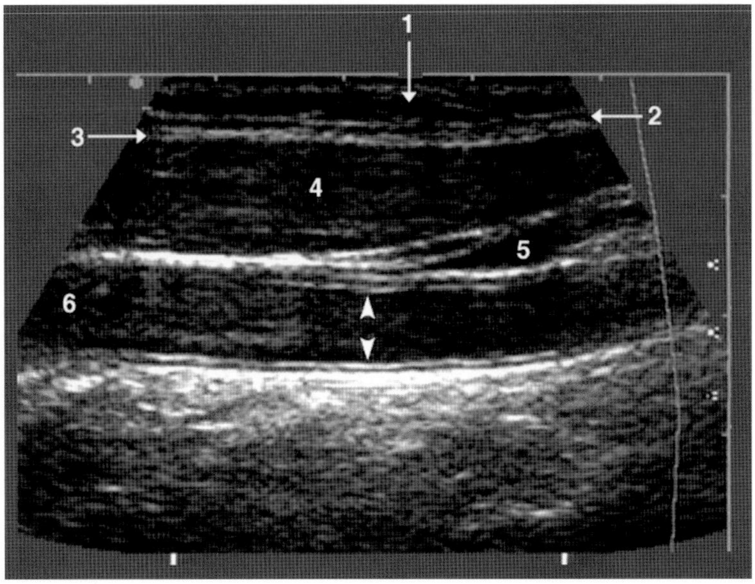

FIGURE 2.5. Right common carotid artery. Lateral view. Longitudinal. Gray scale. *1*, Skin and superficial cervical fascia; *2*, platysma; *3*, deep cervical fascia; *4*, sternocleidomastoid muscle; *5*, jugular vein; *6*, common carotid artery with intima and adventitia.

Diagnosis: Carotid wall structure. The wall of the carotid artery produces parallel echoes corresponding to the adventitial and intimal layers. The hypoechoic region between them represents the media. The intimal reflection does not represent the thickness of the intima, and it should be parallel to the adventitial layer. Visualization of the intimal reflection in longitudinal planes indicates that the image plane passes through the vessel diameter. As shown, this specular reflection is not in the jugular vein wall (2).

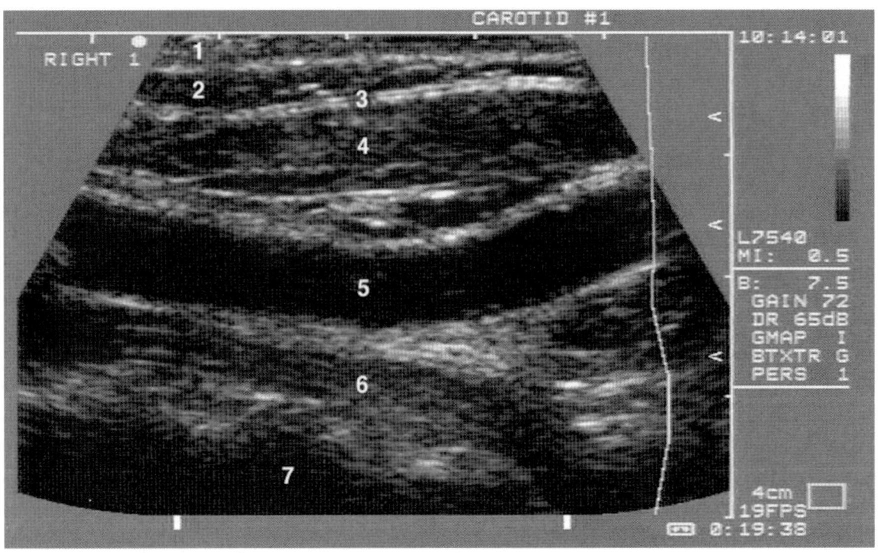

FIGURE 2.6. Right common carotid artery. Anteroposterior view. Longitudinal. Gray scale. *1*, Skin and superficial cervical fascia; *2*, platysma; *3*, deep cervical fascia; *4*, sternocleidomastoid muscle; *5*, right common carotid artery; *6*, longus colli, longus capitis, and scalenus anterior muscles; *7*, transverse process.

Diagnosis: Common carotid artery. Normal anatomy. Anteroposterior view. The right common carotid artery originates from the brachiocephalic trunk, and it is exclusively cervical. The artery is crossed anterolaterally by the omohyoid muscle. Below it, the artery is sited deeply and covered by skin, superficial fascia, platysma, deep cervical fascia, and the sternocleidomastoid, sternohyoid, and sternothyroid muscles. Posteriorly and attached to the fourth to sixth cervical transverse processes are the longus colli, longus capitis, and scalenus anterior muscles (1).

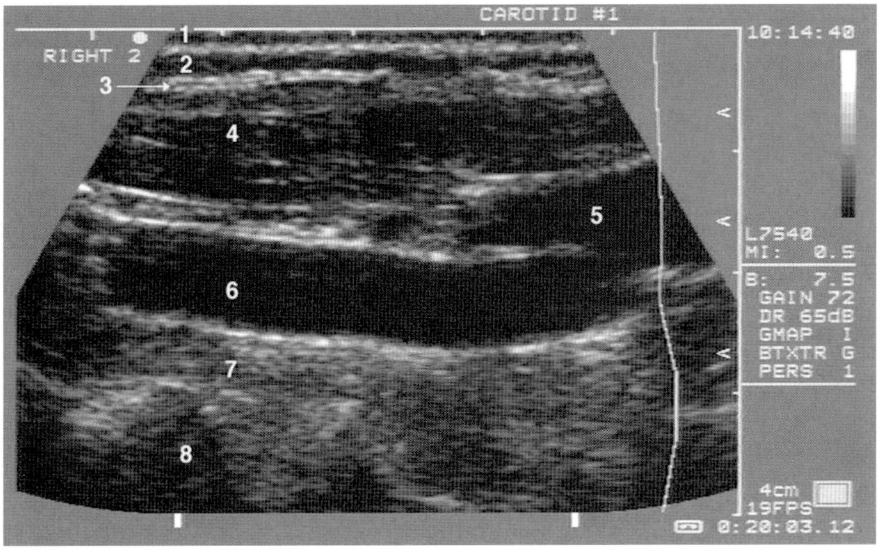

FIGURE 2.7. Right common carotid artery. Lateral view. Longitudinal. Gray scale. *1*, Skin and superficial cervical fascia; *2*, platysma; *3*, deep cervical fascia; *4*, sternocleidomastoid muscle; *5*, right internal jugular vein; *6*, right common carotid artery; *7*, longus colli, longus capitis, and scalenus anterior muscles; *8*, acoustic shadowing resulting from the transverse process of the vertebra.

Diagnosis: Common carotid artery. Normal anatomy. Lateral view. Laterally, the common carotid artery is covered by skin, superficial fascia, platysma, deep fascia, and the medial margin of sternocleidomastoid muscle. The internal jugular vein in the lower neck is lateral and anterior to the common carotid artery (1).

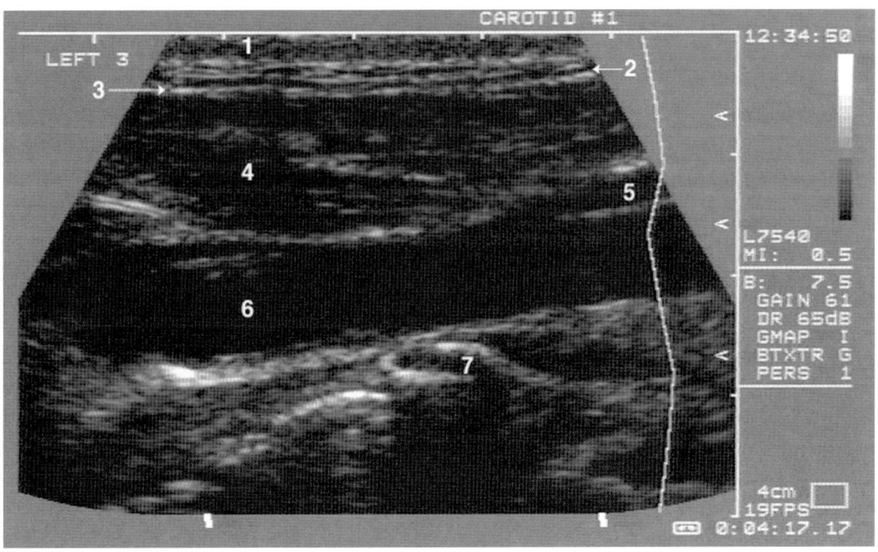

FIGURE 2.8. Left common carotid artery. Posterolateral view. Longitudinal. Gray scale. *1*, Skin and superficial cervical fascia; *2*, platysma; *3*, deep cervical fascia; *4*, sternocleidomastoid muscle; *5*, left internal jugular vein; *6*, left common carotid artery; *7*, laminae of the thyroid cartilage.

Diagnosis: Common carotid artery. Normal anatomy. Posterolateral view. The medial relations of the common carotid artery are the esophagus and trachea and, at a higher level, the larynx and pharynx. The thyroid gland overlaps it anteromedially (1).

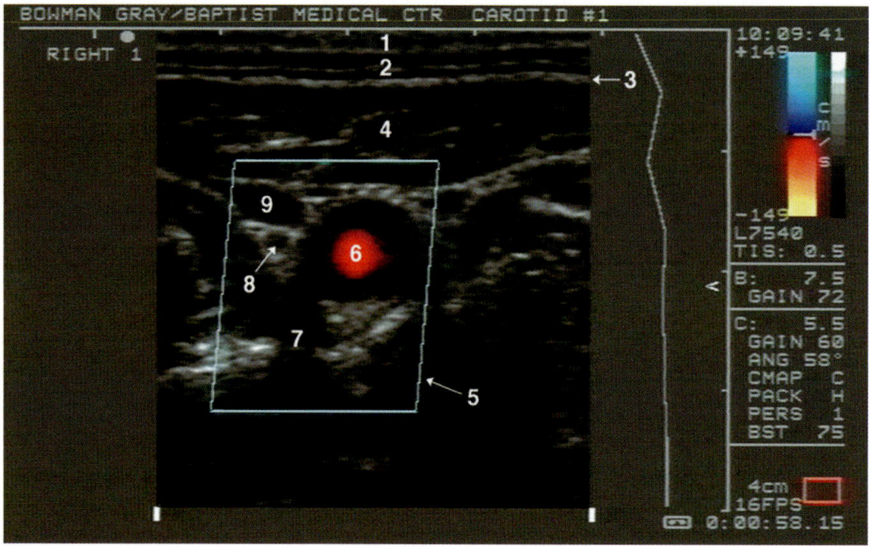

FIGURE 2.9. Right common carotid artery. Transverse view. Color. *1*, Skin and superficial cervical fascia; *2*, platysma; *3*, deep cervical fascia; *4*, sternocleidomastoid muscle; *5*, carotid sheath; *6*, right common carotid artery; *7*, refraction (edge) shadowing; *8*, right vagus nerve; *9*, right internal jugular vein.

Diagnosis: Common carotid artery. Normal anatomy. Transverse view. The carotid sheath is the superior root of the ansa cervicalis. At this level, the vagus nerve is located between and posterior to the internal jugular vein and common carotid artery (3).

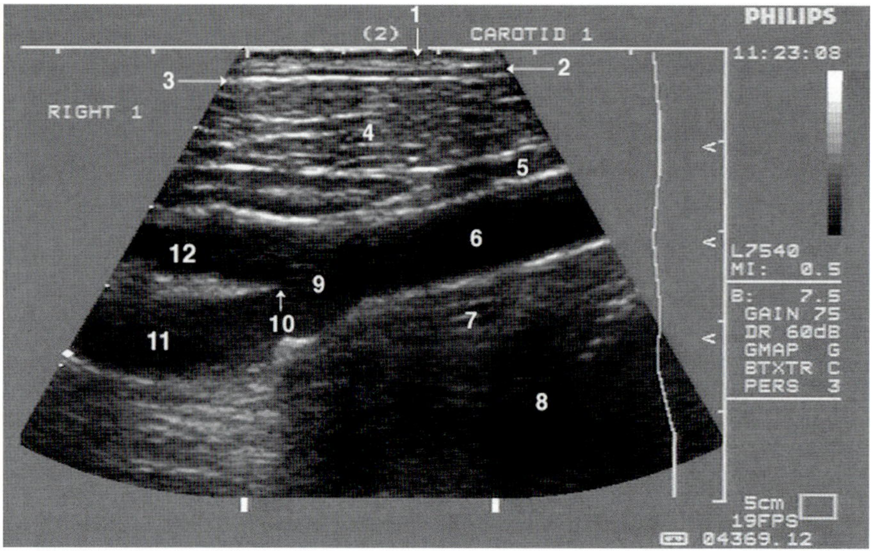

FIGURE 2.10. Bifurcation of the right common carotid artery. Anteroposterior view. Longitudinal. Gray scale. *1*, Skin and superficial cervical fascia; *2*, platysma; *3*, deep cervical fascia; *4*, sternocleidomastoid muscle; *5*, right internal jugular vein; *6*, right common carotid artery; *7*, longus colli, longus capitis, and tendinous slips of scalenus muscle; *8*, transverse process of the vertebra; *9*, bifurcation of the right common carotid artery; *10*, flow divider; *11*, right internal carotid artery with a small plaque at the origin; *12*, right external carotid artery.

Diagnosis: Bifurcation of the common carotid artery. Normal anatomy. Anteroposterior view. The common carotid artery divides into external and internal carotid arteries. At its division, the vessel has a dilatation called the carotid sinus. The carotid sinus usually involves the beginning of the internal carotid artery with thin tunica media and thick tunica adventitia, and containing many baroreceptor endings of the glossopharyngeal nerve (4).

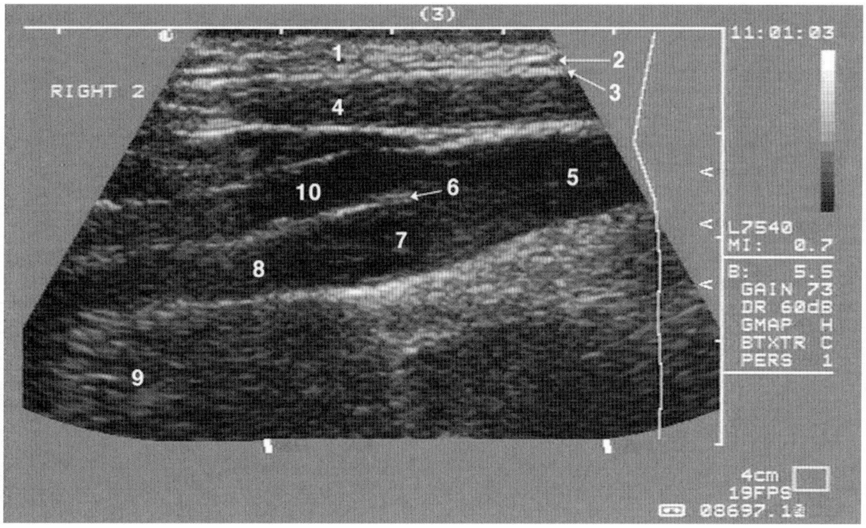

FIGURE 2.11. Bifurcation of the right common carotid artery. Lateral view. Longitudinal. Gray scale. *1*, Skin and superficial cervical fascia; *2*, platysma; *3*, deep cervical fascia; *4*, sternocleidomastoid muscle; *5*, right common carotid artery; *6*, flow divider; *7*, carotid sinus; *8*, right internal carotid artery; *9*, prevertebral soft tissues; *10*, right external carotid artery.

Diagnosis: Bifurcation of the common carotid artery. Normal anatomy. Lateral view. The carotid artery bifurcation is usually located below the level of the hyoid bone and is often related to the larynx. The height of the larynx is age-dependent and, to avoid different heights of division of the common carotid artery according to age, it is more reliable to relate the bifurcation to the vertebral column, usually at the level of C3-4 on the right and at level of C4 on the left (5).

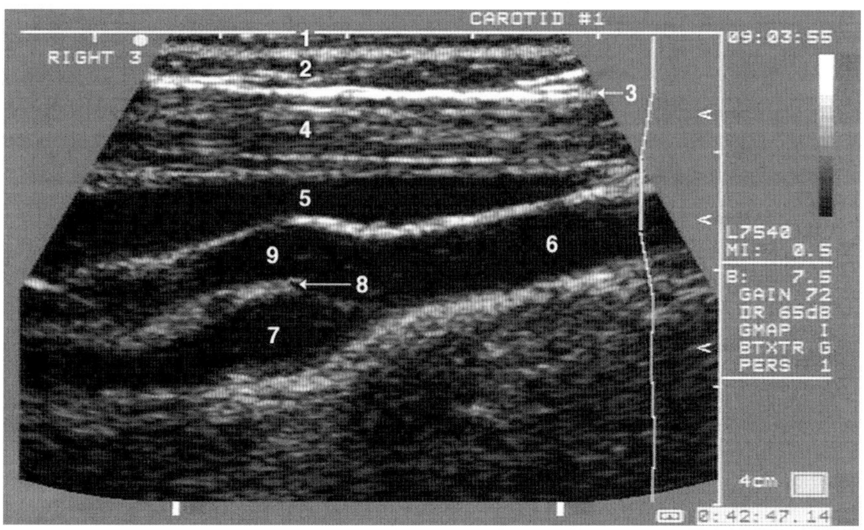

FIGURE 2.12. Bifurcation of the right common carotid artery. Posterolateral view. Longitudinal. Gray scale. *1*, Skin and superficial cervical fascia; *2*, platysma; *3*, deep cervical fascia; *4*, sternocleidomastoid muscle; *5*, right internal jugular vein; *6*, right common carotid artery; *7*, right internal carotid artery, carotid sinus; *8*, flow divider; *9*, right external carotid artery.

Diagnosis: Bifurcation of the common carotid artery. Normal anatomy. Posterolateral view. The origin of the external carotid artery is the third aortic arch, and its precursor arises near the midline. The ultimate position of the external carotid artery is medial or ventral relative to the internal carotid artery (1).

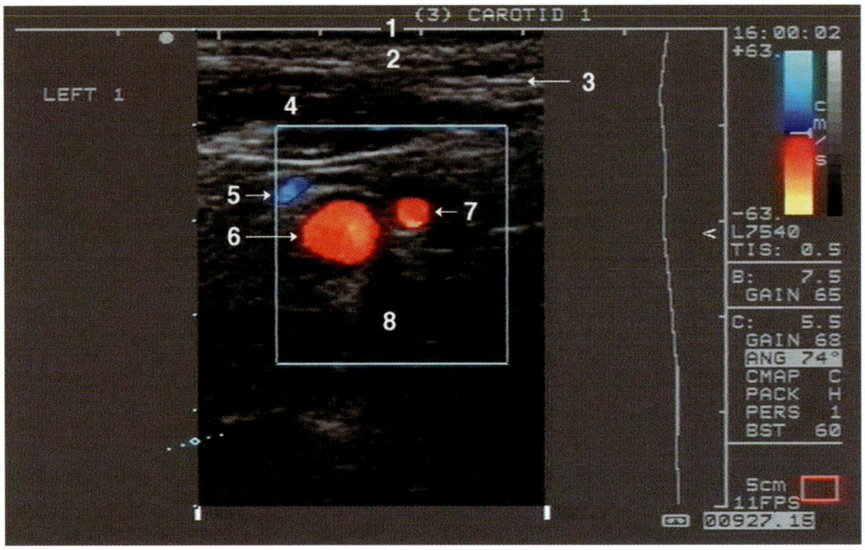

FIGURE 2.13. Bifurcation of the left common carotid artery. Transverse view. Color. *1*, Skin and superficial cervical fascia; *2*, platysma; *3*, deep cervical fascia; *4*, sternocleidomastoid muscle; *5*, left internal jugular vein; *6*, left internal carotid artery; *7*, left external carotid artery; *8*, refraction (edge) shadowing.

Diagnosis: Bifurcation of the common carotid artery. Normal anatomy. Transverse view, color. Color flow imaging can distinguish the internal from the external carotid artery by the simple fact that branches typically arise only from the external carotid artery. The superior thyroidal artery is the first branch that arises usually at the very origin of the external carotid artery from the common carotid. Rarely, the external carotid may arise from the common carotid artery. The internal carotid artery tends to have a larger diameter than the external carotid artery, and the external is usually located anterior and medially with respect to the internal. Because of its high-resistance pattern, the color in the external carotid artery can disappear during diastole. These facts suggest that there should not be any difficulties in identifying and distinguishing these two carotid branches with color flow imaging alone in most normal cases (6).

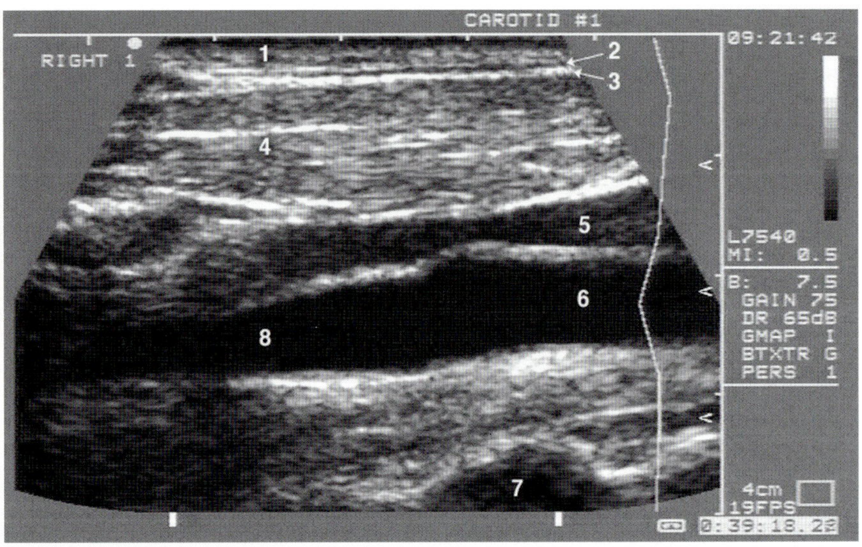

FIGURE 2.14. Right internal carotid artery. Anteroposterior view. Longitudinal. Gray scale. *1*, Skin and superficial cervical fascia; *2*, platysma; *3*, deep cervical fascia; *4*, sternocleidomastoid muscle; *5*, right internal jugular vein; *6*, right common carotid artery; *7*, acoustic shadowing resulting from the transverse process of the vertebra; *8*, right internal carotid artery.

Diagnosis: Internal carotid artery. Normal anatomy. Anteroposterior view. The cervical part of the internal carotid artery has many relations. Posteriorly it adjoins the longus capitis with the superior cervical sympathetic ganglion and superior laryngeal nerve (1).

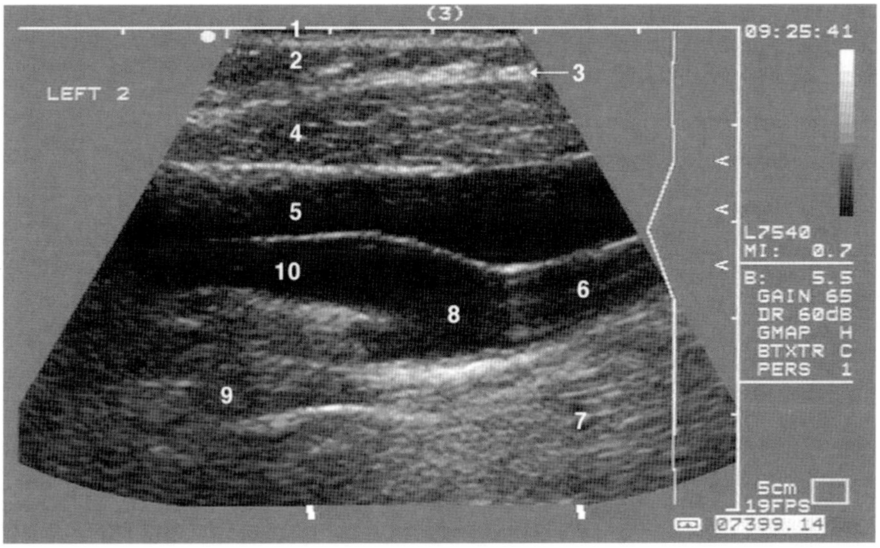

FIGURE 2.15. Left internal carotid artery. Lateral view. Longitudinal. Gray scale. *1*, Skin and superficial cervical fascia; *2*, platysma; *3*, deep cervical fascia; *4*, sternocleidomastoid muscle; *5*, left internal jugular vein; *6*, left common carotid artery; *7*, thyroid gland; *8*, bifurcation of the left common carotid artery; *9*, pharyngeal wall; *10*, left internal carotid artery.

Diagnosis: Internal carotid artery. Normal anatomy. Lateral view. The cervical part of the internal carotid artery begins at the carotid bifurcation and ascends to the carotid canal in the petrous temporal bone. Anteriorly and laterally the internal carotid is covered by the sternocleidomastoid muscle. Except near the skull, the internal jugular vein and the vagus nerve are lateral to the internal carotid artery (1).

A

B

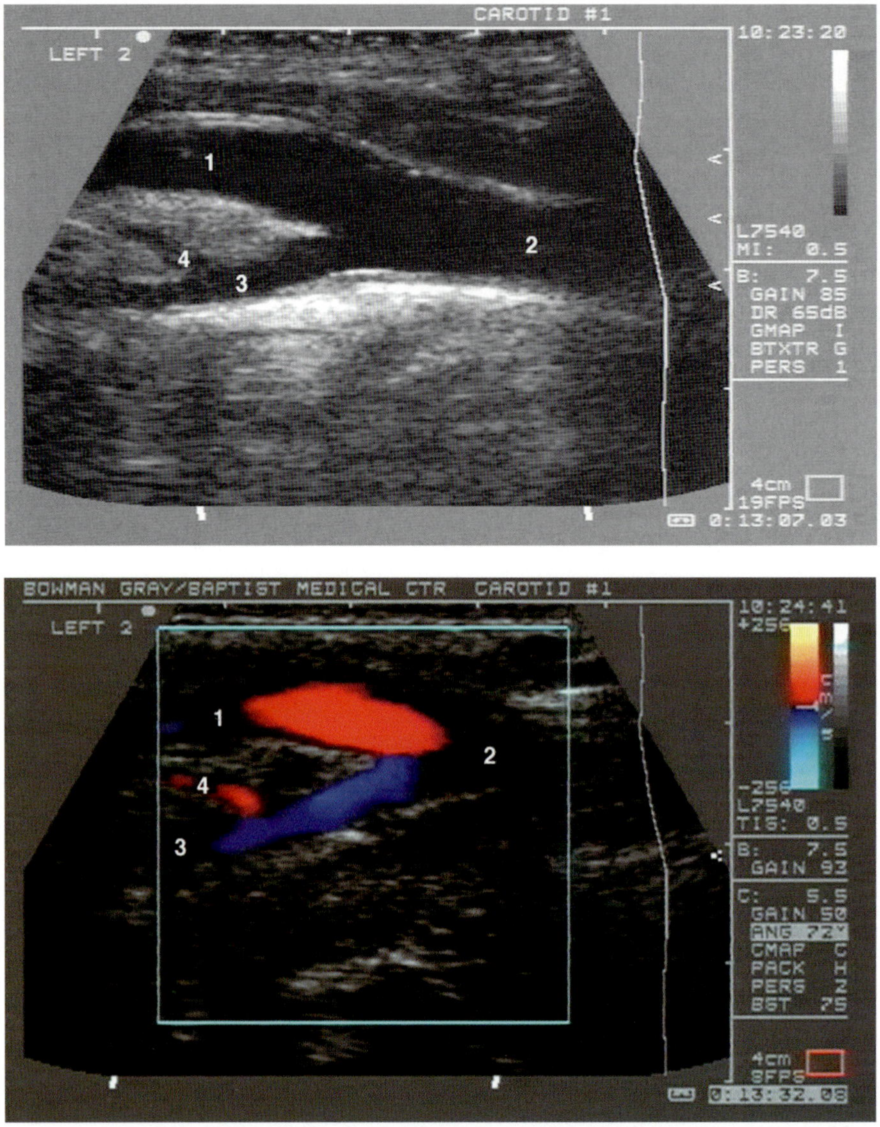

FIGURE 2.16. Left external carotid artery. Lateral view. Longitudinal. Gray scale **(A)** and color **(B)**. Branch of the external carotid artery. *1*, Left internal carotid artery; *2*, left common carotid artery; *3*, left external carotid artery; *4*, branch of the external carotid artery.

Diagnosis: External carotid artery. Normal anatomy. Lateral view. The external carotid artery diminishes rapidly in caliber as a result of its many large branches. Usually the high-resistance pattern of flow in the external carotid artery (ECA) is sufficient to distinguish it from the internal carotid artery. The ECA can be further identified by visualizing its branches, a process made much easier with color flow imaging (7).

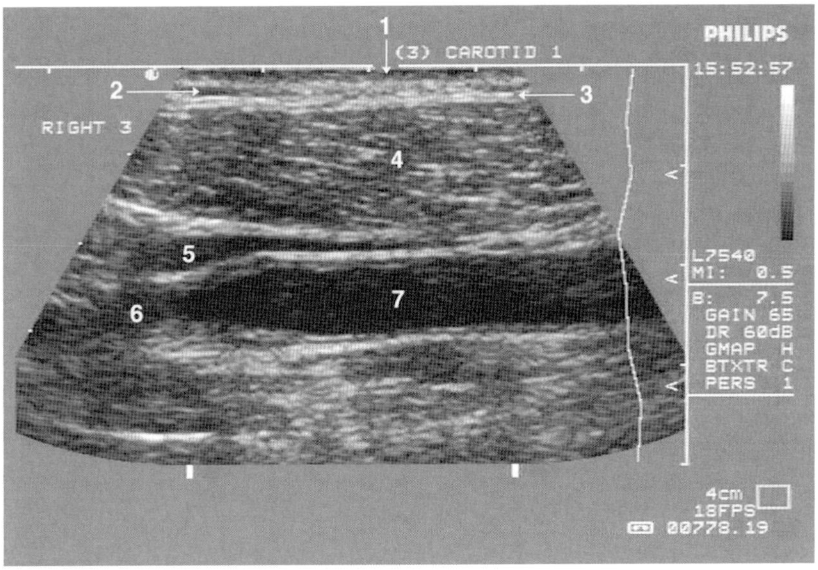

FIGURE 2.17. Right external carotid artery. Posterolateral view. Longitudinal. Gray scale. *1*, Skin and superficial cervical fascia; *2*, platysma; *3*, deep cervical fascia; *4*, sternocleidomastoid muscle; *5*, right internal jugular vein; *6*, right external carotid artery; *7*, right common carotid artery.

Diagnosis: External carotid artery. Normal anatomy. Posterolateral view. At its origin, the external carotid artery lies within the carotid space. At first, it lies medial to the internal carotid artery, but as it ascends in the neck, it passes posterior and laterally. The artery is overlapped in its origin by the anterior border of the sternocleidomastoid. Above this level, the artery is comparatively superficial, being covered by skin, superficial fascia, the cervical branch of the facial nerve, the transverse cutaneous nerve, and the investing layer of deep cervical fascia. The internal jugular vein first lies lateral to the artery and then posterior to it (8).

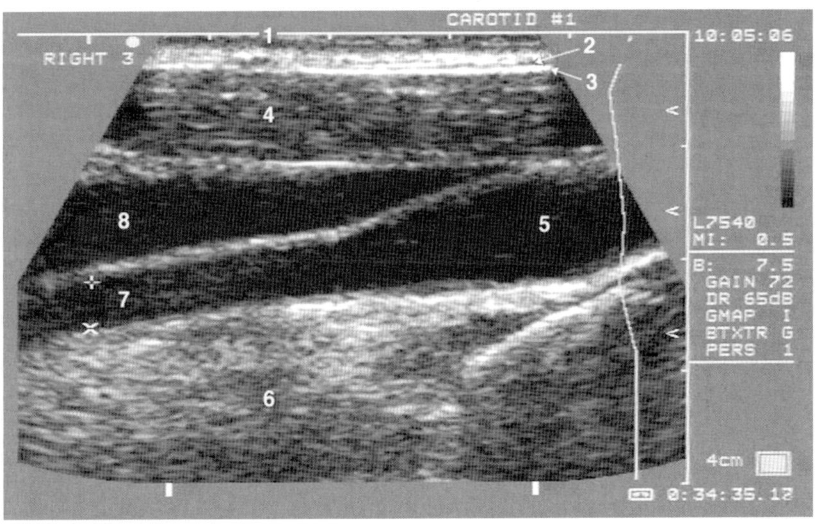

FIGURE 2.18. Right internal carotid artery. Posterolateral view. Longitudinal. Gray scale. *1*, Skin and superficial cervical fascia; *2*, platysma; *3*, deep cervical fascia; *4*, sternocleidomastoid muscle; *5*, carotid sinus; *6*, pharyngeal wall; *7*, right internal carotid artery; *8*, right internal jugular vein.

Diagnosis: Internal carotid artery. Normal anatomy. Posterolateral view. The cervical part of the internal carotid artery presents relatively medially with the pharyngeal wall being separated by fat and pharyngeal veins from the ascending pharyngeal artery and superior laryngeal nerve (1).

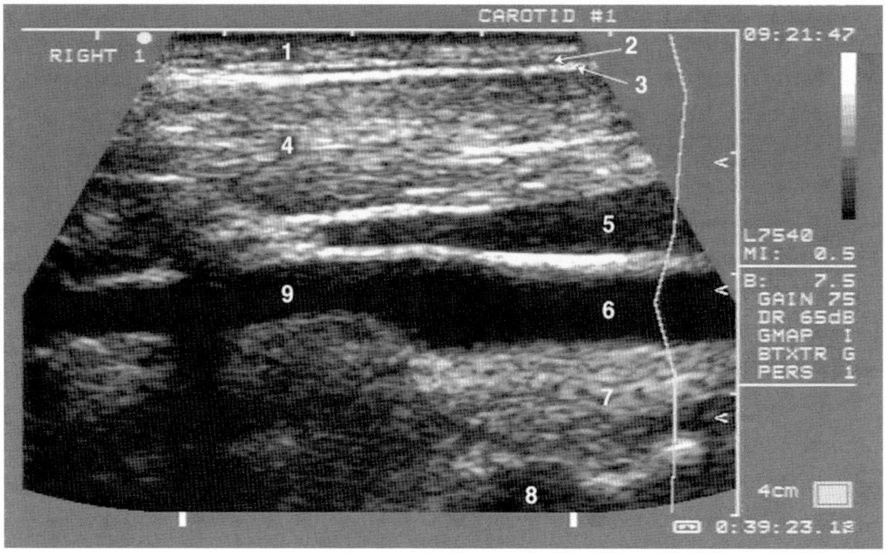

FIGURE 2.19. Right external carotid artery. Anteroposterior view. Longitudinal. Gray scale. *1*, Skin and superficial fascia; *2*, platysma; *3*, deep cervical fascia; *4*, sternocleidomastoid muscle; *5*, right internal jugular vein; *6*, right common carotid artery; *7*, longus colli, longus capitis, and scalenus anterior muscles; *8*, transverse process; *9*, right external carotid artery.

Diagnosis: External carotid artery. Normal anatomy. Anteroposterior view. The external carotid artery is one of the terminal branches of the common carotid artery. It supplies structures in the neck, face, scalp, tongue, and maxilla. The artery typically begins at the level of the upper border of the thyroid cartilage and terminates in the substance of the parotid gland behind the neck of the mandible by dividing into the superficial temporal and maxillary arteries. Superficial to the artery in the carotid space are the skin, superficial fascia, platysma, deep fascia, and the anterior margin of sternocleidomastoid muscle (1).

PEARLS AND PITFALLS

Pearls

- The visualization of the intimal reflection in longitudinal planes indicates that the image plane passes through the vessel diameter.
- At the level of the carotid sheath, the vagus nerve is located between and posterior to the internal jugular vein and common carotid artery.
- Color flow imaging can help distinguish the internal from the external carotid artery because the branches usually arise only from the external carotid artery at the level of the neck.
- The right common carotid artery originates from the brachiocephalic trunk and is exclusively cervical.

Pitfalls

- In 70% of cases, the initial segment of internal carotid artery occupies a lateral-to-posterior position relative to the external carotid artery. When this relationship is reversed, a stenosis of the internal carotid artery can be misinterpreted using continuous wave Doppler alone.
- The height of the larynx is age-dependent, resulting in different heights of division of the common carotid artery. Therefore, the bifurcation should be related to the cervical vertebra.
- If the jugular vein, expanded by Valsalva maneuver, overlies the carotid artery in the beam projection, it will enhance the resolution of the artery, avoiding misdiagnosis in the presence of atherosclerotic changes in the near wall.
- Clinicians should avoid misinterpreting the "intimal reflection" as "intimal thickening," even though the image conveys such an impression.

QUESTIONS

1. Match the three clinically important structures labeled 1, 2, and 3 in Figure 2.20 that are contained in the inferior part of the carotid sheath with the choices below.
   a. Vagus nerve
   b. Common carotid artery
   c. Internal jugular vein

2. Match the branches labeled 1, 2, and 3 in Figure 2.21 shown by color flow imaging at the level of the bifurcation of the left common carotid artery with the choices below.
   a. Superior thyroid artery
   b. Internal carotid artery
   c. External carotid artery

3. Which of the following are branches of the aortic arch?
   a. Right common carotid artery
   b. Right subclavian artery
   c. Left brachiocephalic artery
   d. All of the above
   e. None of the above

4. The right brachiocephalic artery is larger than the left one.
   True or false?

5. Which statement describes the brachiocephalic artery?
   a. It is the shortest branch of the aortic arch.
   b. It is posterior to the manubrium sterni.
   c. It divides into the right subclavian artery and vertebral artery.
   d. All of the above
   e. None of the above

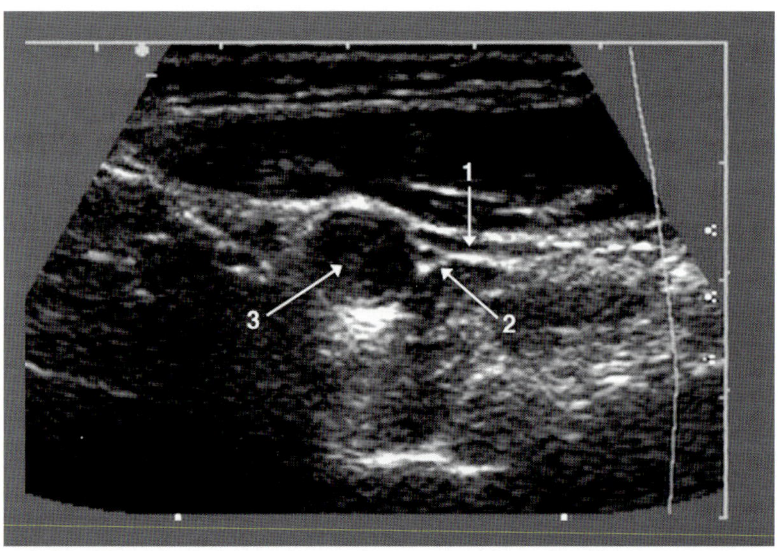

FIGURE 2.20. Right common carotid artery. Transverse view. Gray scale.

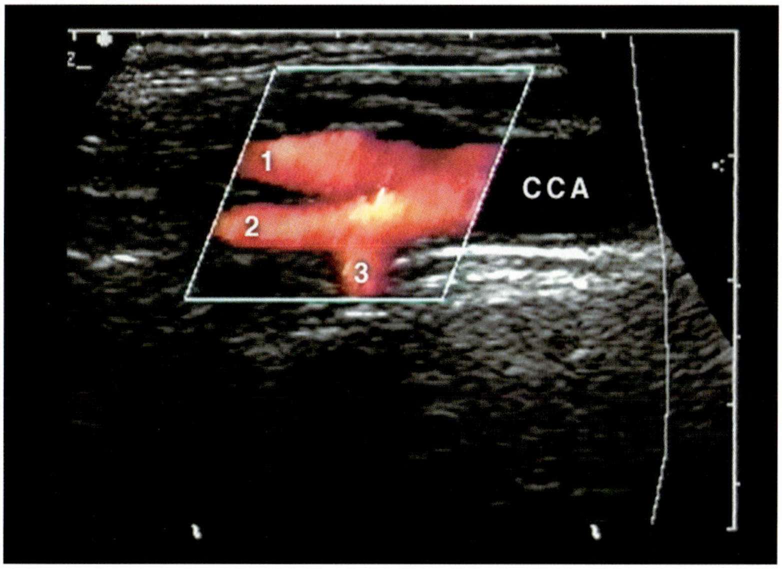

FIGURE 2.21. Left common carotid artery. Lateral view. Longitudinal. Color.

6. The right common carotid artery
   a. arises from the aortic arch.
   b. is the second branch after the subclavian artery.
   c. is exclusively cervical.
   d. a and b
   e. b and c

7. The right common carotid artery originates from the brachiocephalic artery.
   True or false?

8. The internal jugular vein in the lower neck is ________ to the common carotid artery.
   a. anterior
   b. posterior
   c. lateral
   d. a and c
   e. b and c

9. The medial relation(s) of the common carotid artery is/are
   a. the esophagus.
   b. the trachea.
   c. the larynx.
   d. All of the above
   e. None of the above

10. In the carotid sheath, the vagus nerve is located between and posterior to the internal jugular vein and common carotid artery.
   True or false?

11. Which statement is true in relation to the carotid sinus?
    a. It usually involves the beginning of the external carotid artery.
    b. It has a thick tunica media and a thin tunica adventitia.
    c. It contains many baroreceptor endings of the glossopharyngeal nerve.
    d. All of the above
    e. None of the above

12. The bifurcation of the common carotid artery usually
    a. is located above the level of the hyoid bone.
    b. is higher on the right side than on the left.
    c. has the ultimate position of the external carotid artery lateral to the internal carotid artery.
    d. All of the above
    e. None of the above

13. The height of the larynx is age-dependent. To avoid different heights of division of the common carotid artery according to age, it is more reliable to relate the bifurcation to the vertebral column.
    True or false?

14. Color flow imaging with relation to the bifurcation of the common carotid artery can distinguish the internal from the external carotid artery because
    a. branches usually arise only from the external carotid artery.
    b. the internal carotid artery tends to have a larger diameter than the external carotid artery.
    c. its high-resistance pattern causes the color in the external carotid artery to disappear during diastole.
    d. All of the above
    e. None of the above

15. The cervical part of the internal carotid artery has many anatomic relations:
    a. anteriorly and laterally it is covered by sternocleidomastoid muscle.
    b. the internal jugular vein is anterior to the internal carotid artery.
    c. the vagus nerve is medial to the internal carotid artery.
    d. All of the above
    e. None of the above

16. The best way to distinguish the internal carotid artery from the external carotid artery is by the fact that cervical branches arise only from the external carotid artery.
    True or false?

Answers: 1. 1c, 2a, 3b; **2.** 1b, 2c, 3a; **3.** e; **4.** False; **5.** b; **6.** c; **7.** True; **8.** d; **9.** d; **10.** True; **11.** c; **12.** b; **13.** True; **14.** d; **15.** a; **16.** True.

REFERENCES

1. Williams PL. *Gray's anatomy. The anatomical basis of medicine and surgery,* 38th ed. New York: Churchill-Livingstone, 1995.
2. Zwiebel JW. *Introduction to vascular ultrasonography,* 3rd ed. Philadelphia: WB Saunders, 1992.
3. Loes DJ. Neck. In: El-Khonry GY, Bergman RA, Montgomery WJ, eds. *Sectional anatomy by MRI,* 2nd ed. New York: Churchill-Livingstone, 1995.
4. Heath D, Smith P. *The pathology of the carotid body and sinus.* London, UK: Edward Arnold, 1985.
5. Lippert H, Pabst R. *Arterial variations in man. Classification and frequency.* J F Bergmann Verlag. Munchen, 1985.
6. Polak JF. Color flow imaging of the carotid arteries. In: Tegeler CH, Babikian VL, Gomez CR, eds. *Neurosonology.* Chicago: Mosby–Year Book, 1996:68–72.
7. Bluth EI. B-mode evaluation and characterization of carotid plaque. In: Tegeler CH, Babikian VL, Gomez CR, eds. *Neurosonology.* Chicago: Mosby–Year Book, 1996.
8. Snell RS. *Clinical anatomy for medical students,* 5th ed. Boston: Little, Brown, 1995:62–67.

CHAPTER 3

NORMAL HEMODYNAMICS

The word *hemodynamics* is of Greek origin. It is the study and science of blood circulation and the forces and motion of blood flow.

Doppler sonography is a technique for measuring blood flow velocity. A basic understanding of hemodynamics is essential in the interpretation of Doppler signals obtained in clinical practice.

Blood is a fluid. It is a material that can flow and conform to the shape of its container. The term *flow* refers to the volume of blood that moves through a vessel per unit time. Pressure is the first fundamental component of flow. For flow to occur, it is necessary to have a difference in pressure between two areas of the vessel. This is called the *pressure gradient.* The second critical component of flow is resistance. This depends on viscosity, vessel length, and vessel diameter.

Flow is classified as normal, disturbed, or turbulent. The plug and laminar flows are considered to be normal flows. A constant speed of the fluid across the tube is characteristic of the former and a parabolic shape describes the latter. Disturbed flow occurs when the parallel streamlines that characterize normal flow are disturbed. Turbulent flow is random and chaotic.

The time dependence of blood flow velocity on cardiac activity is described by the flow waveform. The effect of vessel geometry on spectral Doppler waveform is known.

This chapter illustrates hemodynamic principles to recognize normal flow patterns seen in the aortic arch and carotid system.

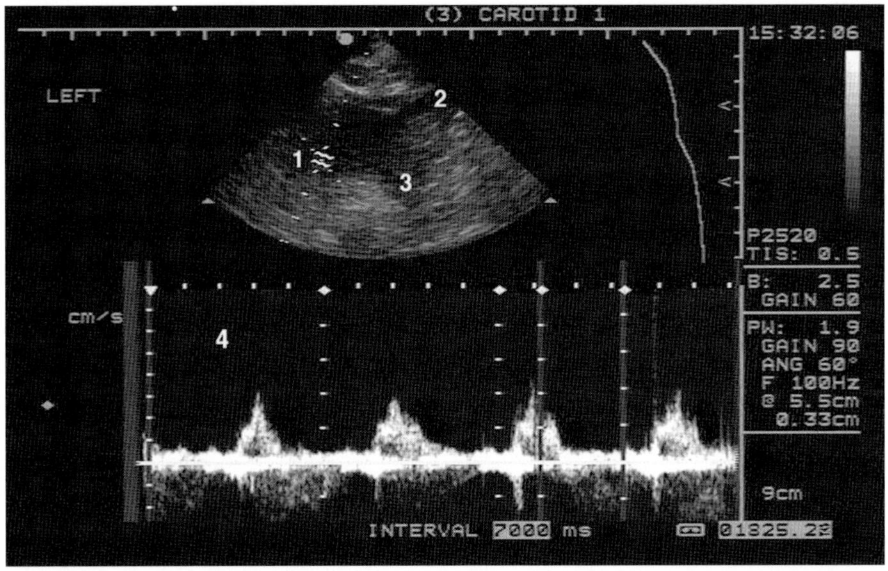

A

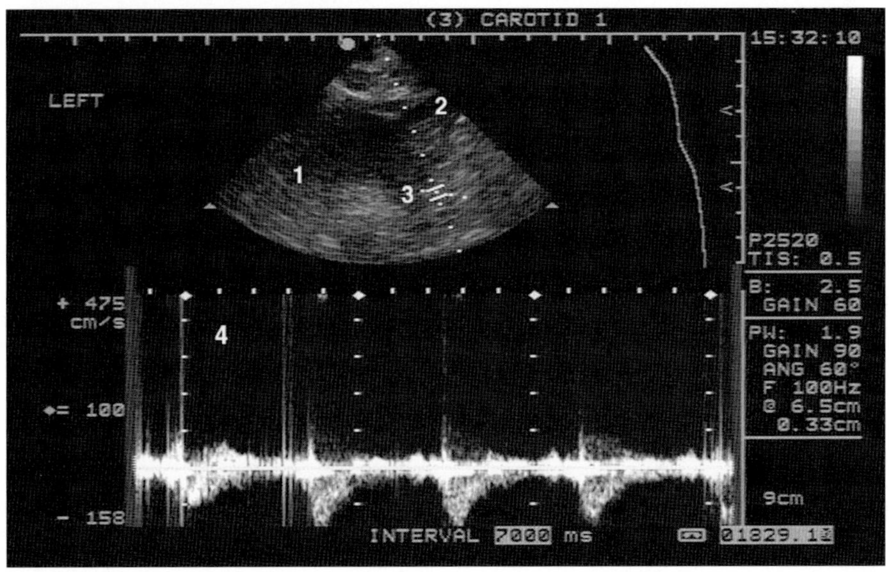

B

FIGURE 3.1. A: Ascending aorta through suprasternal notch. Gray scale. Doppler spectral waveform. *1,* Ascending aorta; *2,* origin of the left common carotid artery or left subclavian artery; *3,* descending aorta; *4,* Doppler spectrum of the ascending aorta. **B:** Descending aorta through suprasternal notch. Gray scale. Doppler spectral waveform. *1,* Ascending aorta; *2,* origin of the left common carotid artery or left subclavian artery; *3,* descending aorta; *4,* Doppler spectrum of the descending aorta.

Diagnosis: Aortic arch. Normal Doppler waveform. In patients with normal aortic valves, antegrade systolic flow toward the transducer in the ascending aorta is seen, and there is either minimal early diastolic reversal or no retrograde flow. In the descending aorta, the flow wave becomes more rounded than in the ascending aorta and the incisura becomes inapparent with spectral broadening in both (1).

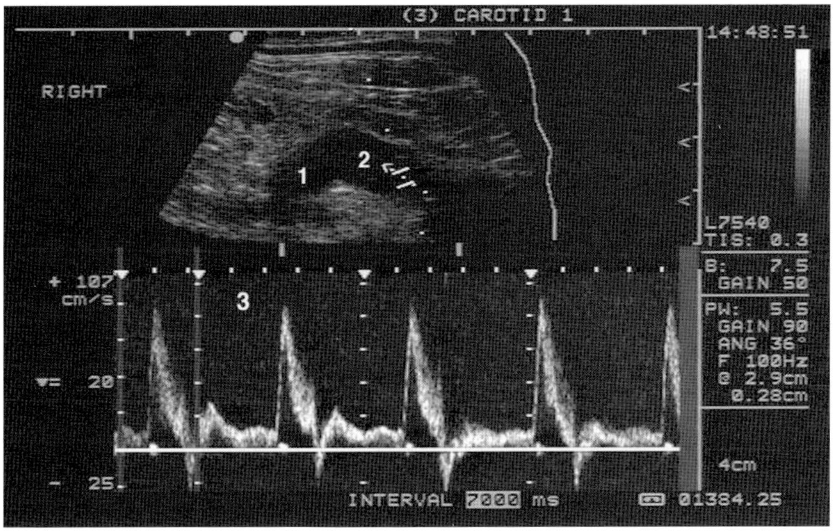

FIGURE 3.2. Right brachiocephalic artery. Anteroposterior view. Longitudinal. Gray scale. Doppler spectral waveform. *1,* Right subclavian artery; *2,* brachiocephalic artery; *3,* Doppler spectrum of the brachiocephalic artery.

Diagnosis: Brachiocephalic artery. Normal Doppler spectrum. The brachiocephalic artery shows a high-resistance flow pattern with a large positive deflection in systole, a period of flow reversal, and lesser positive deflection in diastole. Because of the three components, it is called *triphasic* (2).

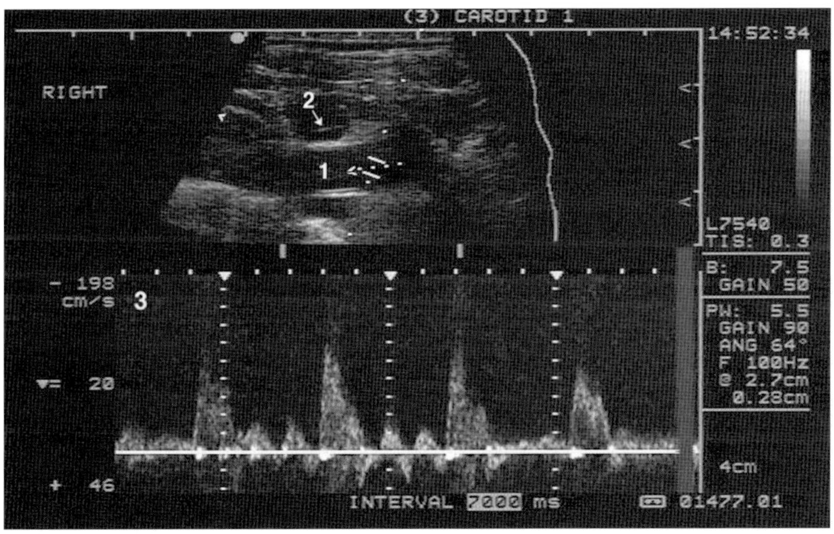

FIGURE 3.3. Right subclavian artery. Longitudinal. Gray scale. Doppler spectral waveform. *1,* Right subclavian artery; *2,* right internal jugular vein and internal jugular valve; *3,* Doppler spectrum of the right subclavian artery.

Diagnosis: Subclavian artery. Normal Doppler spectrum. The brachiocephalic artery is the first major artery to arise from the aortic arch on the right side. The subclavian artery arises from the brachiocephalic artery. It can be insonated by placing the probe in the supraclavicular fossa, showing a normal triphasic signal. Diastolic oscillations in the spectrum after tapping the brachial artery are observed.

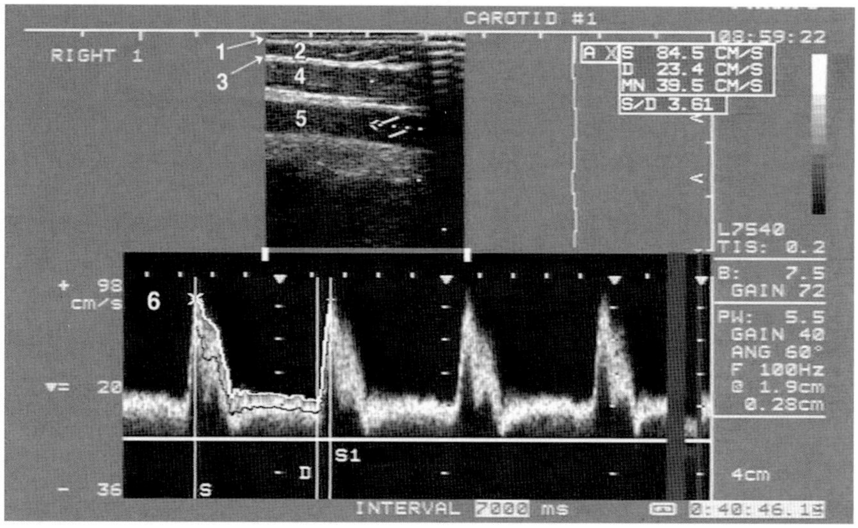

FIGURE 3.4. Right common carotid artery. Anteroposterior view. Longitudinal. Gray scale. Doppler spectrum. *1,* Skin and superficial cervical fascia; *2,* platysma; *3,* deep cervical fascia; *4,* sternocleidomastoid muscle; *5,* right common carotid artery; *6,* Doppler spectrum of the right common carotid artery.

Diagnosis: Common carotid artery. Normal Doppler spectrum. The normal common carotid Doppler spectrum is intermediate between the internal and the external carotid signals. There is a less rapid drop-off in diastole than in the external signal but not as gradual as in the internal signal. It has a clearly defined envelope and an uncluttered spectral window with narrow spectral width (4).

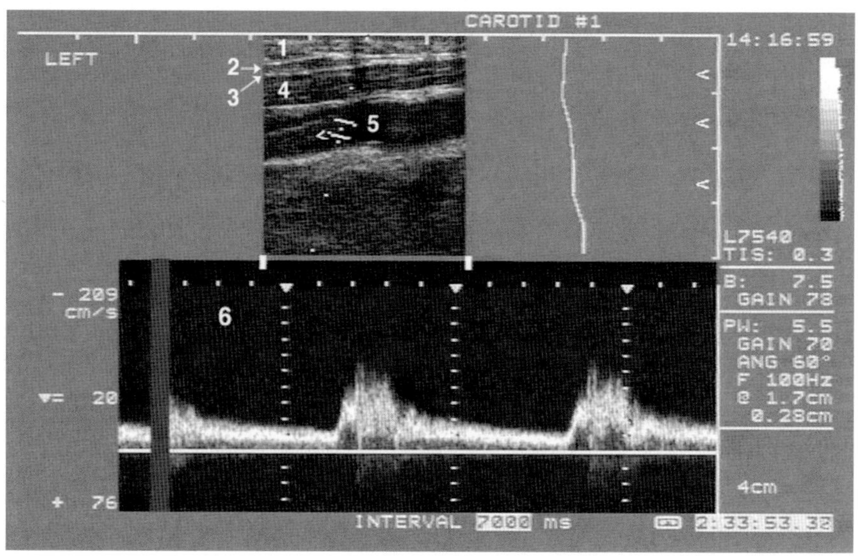

FIGURE 3.5. Bifurcation of the left common carotid artery. Lateral view. Longitudinal. Gray scale. Doppler spectrum. *1,* Skin and superficial cervical fascia; *2,* platysma; *3,* deep cervical fascia; *4,* sternocleidomastoid muscle; *5,* bifurcation of the left common carotid artery; *6,* Doppler spectrum of the left common carotid bifurcation.

Diagnosis: Bifurcation of the common carotid artery. Normal Doppler spectrum. Some mild turbulence or flow disturbance may occur within the bulb area around the bifurcation, which is normal. It is inherent to the flow of the carotid bifurcation (5).

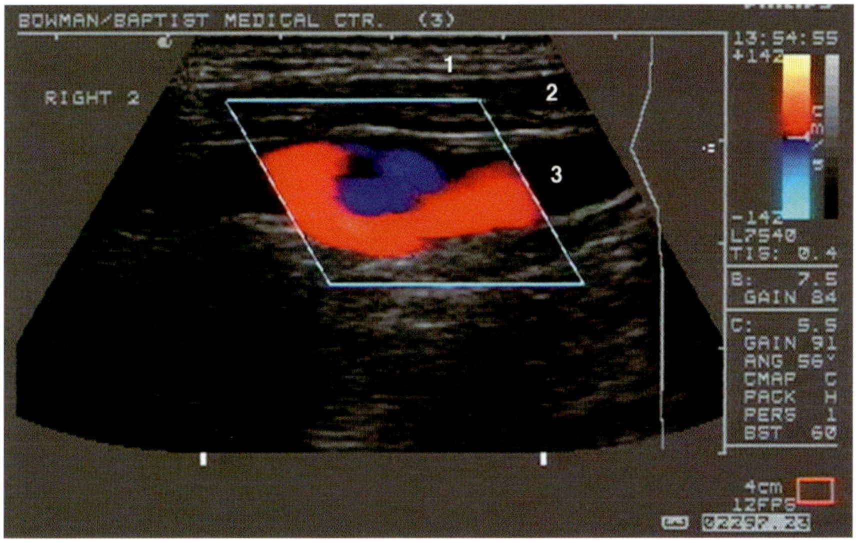

FIGURE 3.6. Bifurcation of the right common carotid artery. Lateral view. Longitudinal. Color flow imaging. *1*, Skin, superficial cervical fascia, and platysma; *2*, sternocleidomastoid muscle; *3*, right common carotid artery and bifurcation. *Red,* antegrade flow; *blue*, retrograde flow.

Diagnosis: Normal bifurcation of the common carotid artery. Color flow imaging. Color flow imaging typically shows a zone of flow reversal in the distal common carotid opposite to the flow divider between the internal and external carotid arteries (6).

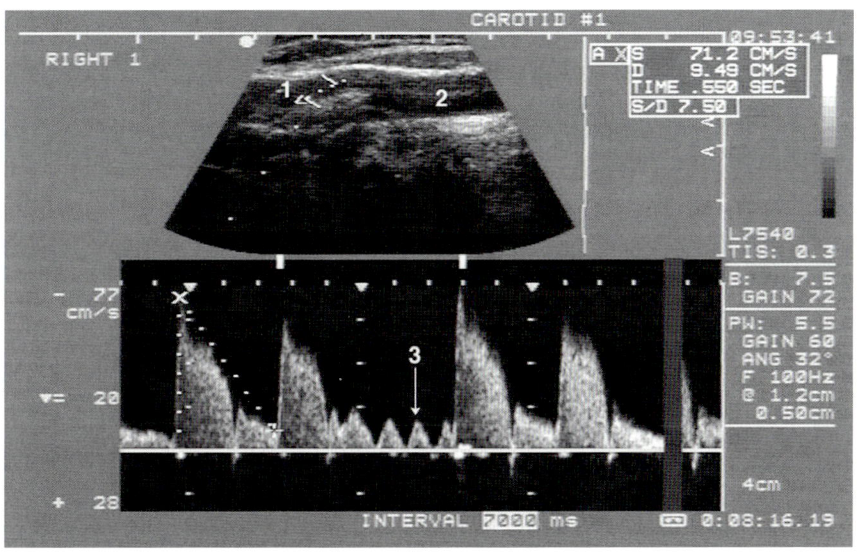

FIGURE 3.7. Right external carotid artery. Anteroposterior view. Longitudinal. Gray scale. Doppler spectrum. *1*, Right external carotid artery; *2*, right common carotid artery; *3*, diastolic oscillations from the temporal artery tap maneuver.

Diagnosis: External carotid artery. Normal Doppler spectrum. This case demonstrates the typical high-resistance waveform of the external carotid artery with diastolic oscillations from the temporal artery tap maneuver. These waveform oscillations can be found beyond the external carotid artery in the common carotid artery as well as in the internal carotid artery. The temporal tap alone may not reliably distinguish the external carotid artery from the internal or common carotid arteries (7).

PEARLS AND PITFALLS

Pearls

- The brachiocephalic and subclavian arteries show a high-resistance flow pattern with three components: a large positive deflection in systole, a period of flow reversal, and a lesser positive deflection in diastole.
- Mild turbulence occurs at the outer wall of all carotid bulbs. This hemodynamic pattern is characteristic for normal carotid bifurcations.
- Diastolic oscillations that appear in the Doppler waveform of the external carotid artery from the temporal tap maneuver are not enough alone to distinguish the external carotid artery from the internal or common carotid arteries.
- Even though the curve of the aortic arch causes a dramatic change in the initial Doppler waveform, the complex flow associated with the bend and disparate distal vascular impedance must not be considered as turbulent flow.

Pitfalls

- The absence of flow separation in the carotid bulb area may be associated with underlying vascular changes of anatomy because the internal carotid artery originated directly from the common carotid artery without common or internal carotid bulb. This may lead the clinician to misdiagnose early atherosclerosis in the carotid bulb.
- The presence of flow separation does not exclude atherosclerotic disease in the bifurcation if the plaque is located at the flow divider.
- It is impossible to assess progression or regression of nonstenotic plaques based only on the Doppler spectrum because flow separation may confuse analysis.
- A common error is to believe that the plug or parabolic flow is the only form of laminar flow. The natural, pulsatile, helical flow in arteries is a form of laminar flow.

QUESTIONS

1. The pattern of blood flow in the aorta differs with the level at which the vessel is scanned. The spectral broadening in the ascending and descending aorta means there is laminar flow.

   True or false?

2. The period of net flow reversal to the negative side of the zero line results from the ________ of the vascular bed in the extremities.
   a. high resistance
   b. low resistance
   c. medium resistance
   d. All of the above
   e. None of the above

3. A flow pattern with a large positive deflection in systole, a period of flow reversal, and lesser positive deflection in diastole is called
   a. monophasic.
   b. biphasic.
   c. triphasic.
   d. All of the above
   e. None of the above

4. The normal Doppler spectrum of the left brachiocephalic artery is a high-resistance flow pattern.

   True or false?

5. After tapping the brachial artery during the duplex scanning of the subclavian artery, one can observe
   a. an audible signal in the artery being examined.
   b. a visible signal in the Doppler spectrum of the subclavian artery.
   c. All of the above
   d. None of the above
   e. No change.

6. The subclavian artery arises from the
   a. brachiocephalic artery.
   b. aortic arch.
   c. vertebral artery.
   d. a and b
   e. b and c

7. The brachiocephalic artery Doppler spectral waveform is called "triphasic" because it is a high-resistance flow pattern.

   True or false?

8. The subclavian artery
   a. has a low-resistance flow pattern.
   b. shows an abnormal triphasic signal.
   c. arises on the right side from the aortic arch.
   d. All of the above
   e. None of the above

9. The normal common carotid artery Doppler spectrum shows a clearly defined envelope and a narrow spectral width.
   True or false?

10. The normal common carotid artery Doppler spectrum is
   a. equal to the internal carotid artery.
   b. equal to the external carotid artery.
   c. intermediate between the internal and the external carotid arteries.
   d. All of the above
   e. None of the above

11. The clearly defined envelope and narrow spectral width of the Doppler spectrum of the common carotid artery relates to
   a. laminar flow.
   b. parabolic flow.
   c. plug flow.
   d. a and b
   e. b and c

12. The presence of mild turbulence in the bulb area around the bifurcation indicates
   a. flow disturbance.
   b. a normal occurrence in the bulb area.
   c. an inherent occurrence of the carotid bifurcation.
   d. All of the above
   e. None of the above

13. Flow reversal with color flow imaging at the bifurcation of the common carotid artery indicates an early sign of arteriosclerosis.
   True or false?

14. The diastolic oscillations that appear in the high-resistance waveform of the external carotid artery from the temporal tap maneuver ________ distinguish it from the internal or common carotid arteries.
   a. may not reliably
   b. may reliably
   c. always
   d. never
   e. is enough alone to

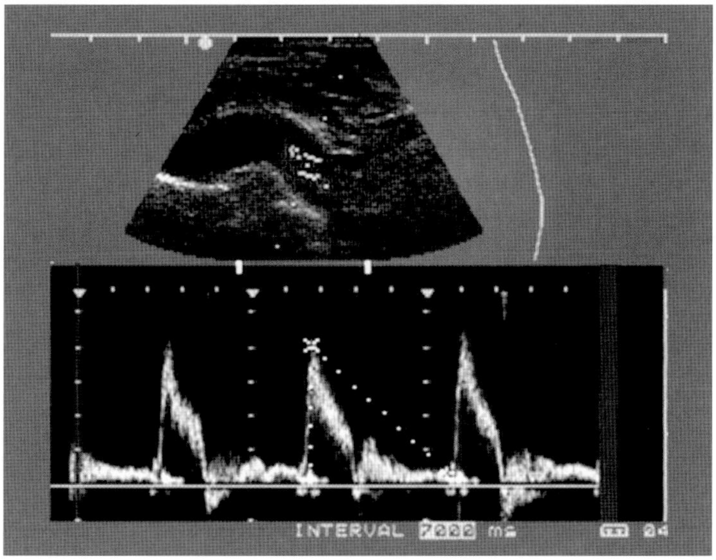

FIGURE 3.8.

15. The flow pattern shown in Figure 3.8 is
    a. a high-resistance flow pattern.
    b. called a "triphasic" waveform.
    c. the normal spectrum found in the brachiocephalic artery.
    d. All of the above
    e. None of the above

16. Figure 3.9. The diastolic oscillations (1) that appear after temporal artery tap maneuver imply that the Doppler spectrum corresponds to the external carotid artery.

True or false?

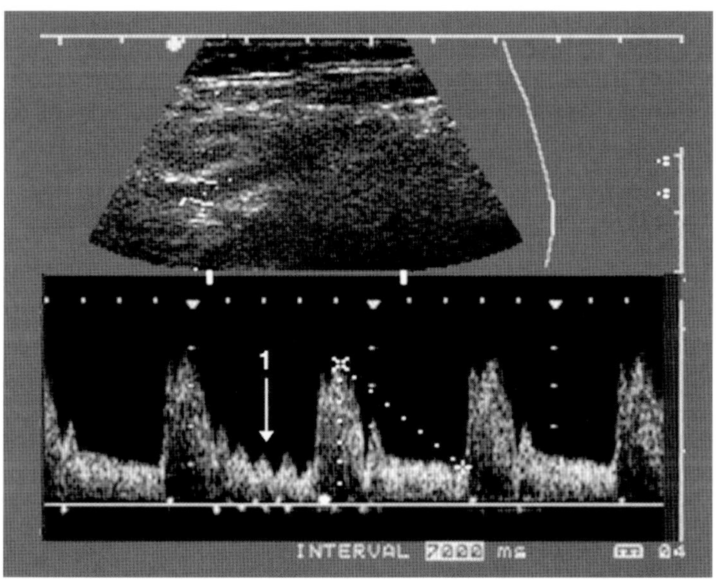

FIGURE 3.9.

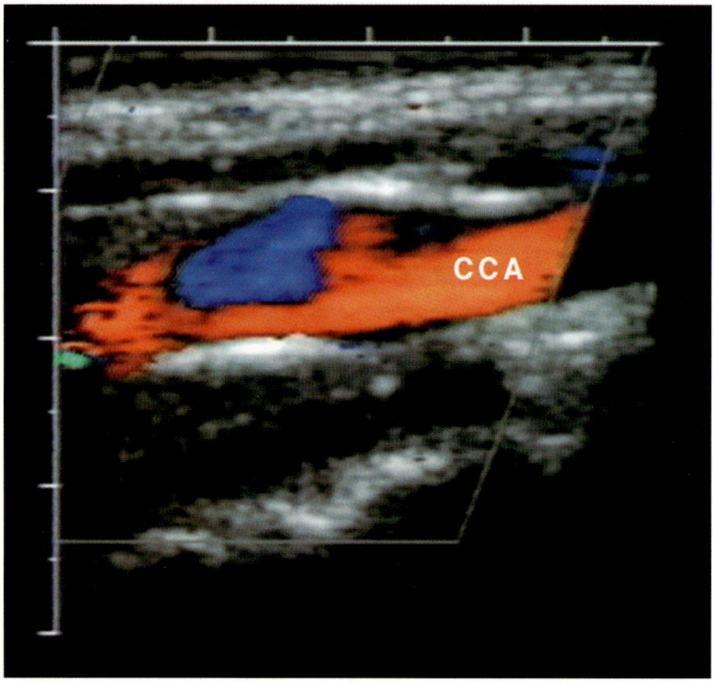

FIGURE 3.10. Right bifurcation of the common carotid artery. Longitudinal view. Color.

17. In this longitudinal view of the right bifurcation with color flow imaging (Fig. 3.10),
    a. the blue "island" within the red blood flow consists of flow reversal.
    b. the blue "island" appears in healthy subjects.
    c. the blue "island" is located opposite the flow divider.
    d. All of the above
    e. None of the above

Answers: **1.** False; **2.** a; **3.** c; **4.** False; **5.** c; **6.** d; **7.** False; **8.** e; **9.** True; **10.** c; **11.** d; **12.** d; **13.** False; **14.** a; **15.** d; **16.** False; **17.** d.

REFERENCES

1. O'Rourke MF. Pressure and flow waves in systemic arteries and the anatomical design of the arterial system. *J Appl Physiol* 1967;23:139–149.
2. Barnes RW, Wilson MR. *Doppler ultrasonic evaluation of peripheral arterial disease: a programmed audiovisual instruction.* Iowa City, IA: University of Iowa Press, 1976.
3. Edwards JM, Zierler RE. Duplex ultrasound assessment of upper extremity arteries. In: Zwiebel WJ, ed. *Introduction to vascular ultrasonography,* 3rd ed. Philadelphia: WB Saunders, 1992.
4. Zwiebel WJ, Knighton R. Duplex examination of the carotid arteries. *Semin Ultrasound CT MR* 1990;11:123.
5. Ku DN, Giddens DP, Zarins CK, et al. Pulsatile flow and atherosclerosis in the human carotid bifurcation: positive correlation between plaque location and low oscillating shear stress. *Arteriosclerosis* 1985:5:209–302.
6. Middleton WD, Foley WD, Lawson TL. Flow reversal in the normal carotid bifurcation: color Doppler flow imaging analysis. *Radiology* 1988;167:207–210.
7. Kliewer MA, Freed KS, Hertzberg BS. Temporal artery tap: usefulness and limitations in carotid sonography. *Radiology* 1996;201:481–484.

CHAPTER 4

CAROTID SYSTEM PATHOLOGY

The relationship between large-vessel extracranial atherothrombosis, cardiac or aortic disease, intracranial small-vessel disease, transient ischemic attacks, and cerebral infarction is well known. Embolism, hemodynamic compromise, or a combination of both is the mechanism for cerebral ischemic events.

The principal role of duplex carotid examination is in the detection of stenotic or occlusive lesions of the carotid system. Of particular concern is the accurate diagnosis of critical stenosis, which is associated with increased risk of cerebral infarction. A carotid lesion that causes more than 75% diameter narrowing is defined as *critical stenosis* and is associated with increased risk of cerebral infarction. Information about plaque composition is also helpful in selecting patients for surgical or medical therapy.

Doppler ultrasound studies can define the grade of carotid stenosis and assess collateral flow. Real time B-mode ultrasonography can detect plaque and nonobstructive ulcerated plaque in the carotid system. Color flow imaging allows a rapid documentation of the presence and direction of flow, an accurate estimation of the angle of insonation, greater accuracy in locating the region of highest flow velocity, increased identification of surface features of the plaques, and higher accuracy in the diagnosis of near occlusion.

The criteria for grading carotid artery stenosis as well as the advantages of color-coded Doppler sonography in the evaluation of different pathologic conditions of the extracranial carotid system are demonstrated in this chapter.

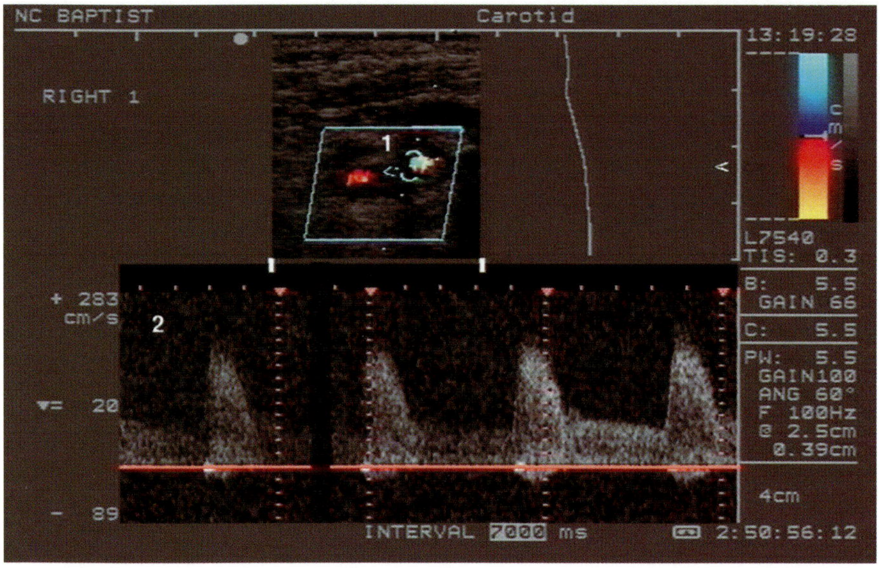

FIGURE 4.1. Right internal carotid artery. Anteroposterior view. Longitudinal. Color. Doppler spectrum. *1*, Sample was placed in the right internal carotid artery; *2*, Doppler spectrum showing peak systolic velocity of 204 cm/s and end diastolic velocity of 60 cm/s.

Diagnosis: Internal carotid stenosis. The hemodynamic assessment with Doppler sonography forms the foundation for detection of carotid stenosis. The key parameters for interpretation are the peak systolic and end diastolic velocities. Several other parameters including the internal carotid artery to common carotid artery velocity ratio or the presence of extensive plaque on B-mode imaging provide adjunctive information (1).

TABLE 4.1. GRADING OF CAROTID ARTERY STENOSIS WITH DUPLEX SONOGRAPHY (WAKE FOREST UNIVERSITY SCHOOL OF MEDICINE CRITERIA)

Degree Stenosis	Peak Systolic Velocity (ICA)	End Diastolic Velocity (ICA)	ICA/CCA Ratio
0%–49%	<140 cm/s	<40 cm/s	<2
50%–74%	>140 cm/s	<125 cm/s	>2
75%–94%	>140 cm/s	>125 cm/s	>3
95%–99%	Variable	Variable	Variable
Occlusion	No flow	No flow	—

Abbreviations: CCA, common carotid artery; ICA, internal carotid artery.

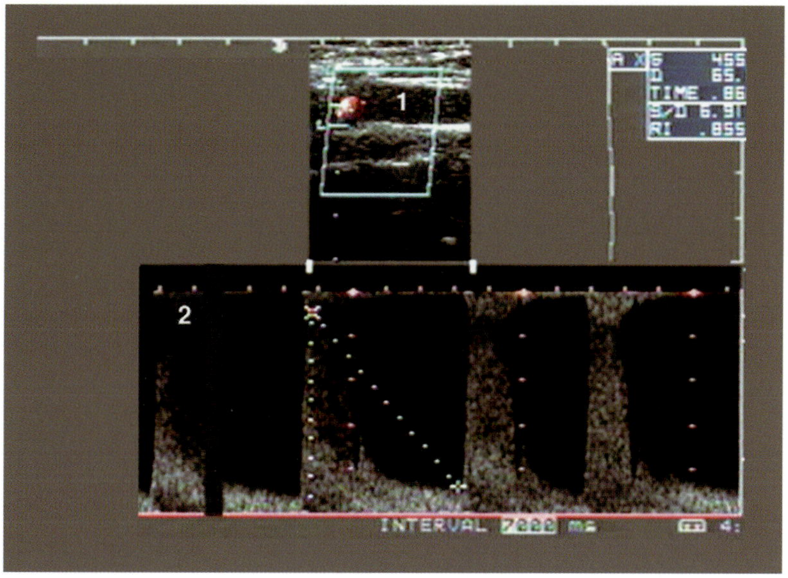

FIGURE 4.2. Left external carotid artery. Lateral view. Longitudinal. Color. Doppler spectrum. *1*, Sample volume places in the left external carotid artery; *2*, Doppler spectrum of the external carotid artery shows peak systolic velocity of 455 cm/s and end diastolic velocity of 65 cm/s.

Diagnosis: External carotid artery stenosis. Carotid ultrasound is usually performed to evaluate plaque and stenosis in the carotid bifurcation, especially in the internal carotid artery (ICA). External carotid artery (ECA) stenosis is less frequent and clinically less important than ICA stenosis, but it may be the cause of carotid bruit. Branches of the ECA may serve as critical collateral pathways to the cerebral hemisphere when the internal carotid is occluded. The Doppler criteria concerning external carotid stenosis are the same as for internal carotid stenosis. The cardinal Doppler parameters for stenosis measurement, such as peak systolic velocity, peak end diastolic velocity, the systolic velocity ratio, and the diastolic velocity ratio, have been studied to establish their accuracy. Only in severe stenosis is the peak systolic velocity and its ratio to the systolic velocity of the common carotid artery reliable to define the grade of stenosis (2).

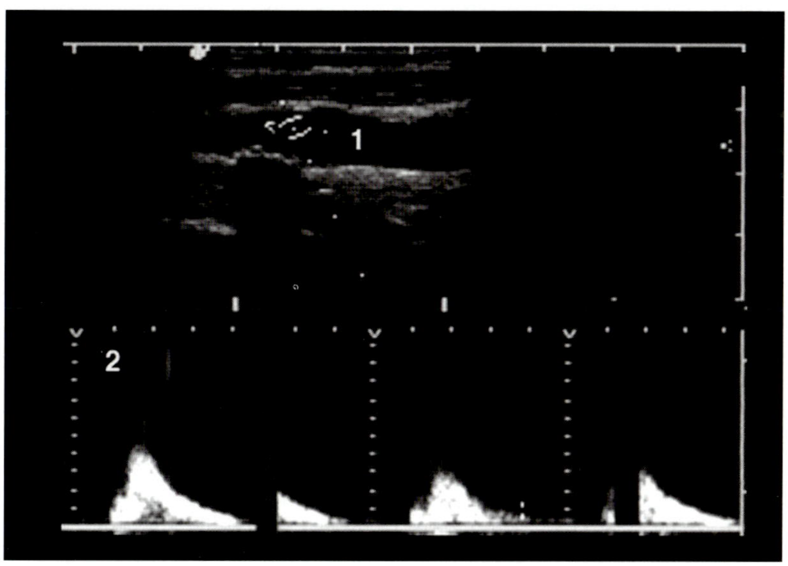

FIGURE 4.3. Right common carotid artery. Lateral view. Longitudinal. Gray scale and Doppler spectrum. *1*, Sample volume placed at the bifurcation of the right common carotid artery; *2*, Doppler spectrum was sampled at a point proximal to a high-grade stenosis.

Diagnosis: Pulsatility interpretation. If the internal carotid artery is severely obstructed or occluded, then the common carotid artery waveform proximal to that point exhibits high-pulsatility features. To avoid sources of error, the simplest and most effective method to interpret common carotid pulsatility is to compare the waveforms recorded over both common carotid arteries. Care must be taken during the visual interpretation of carotid waveforms because the overall status of the cardiovascular system may affect the waveform configuration. Increased pulsatility in the absence of carotid obstruction is seen with hypertension, tachycardia, and diminished arterial compliance caused by distal vascular disease, as in the case shown in which there is mostly antegrade flow, despite the loss of diastolic flow. The asymmetry of waveform is the key to avoiding a false-positive diagnosis of distal carotid obstruction (3).

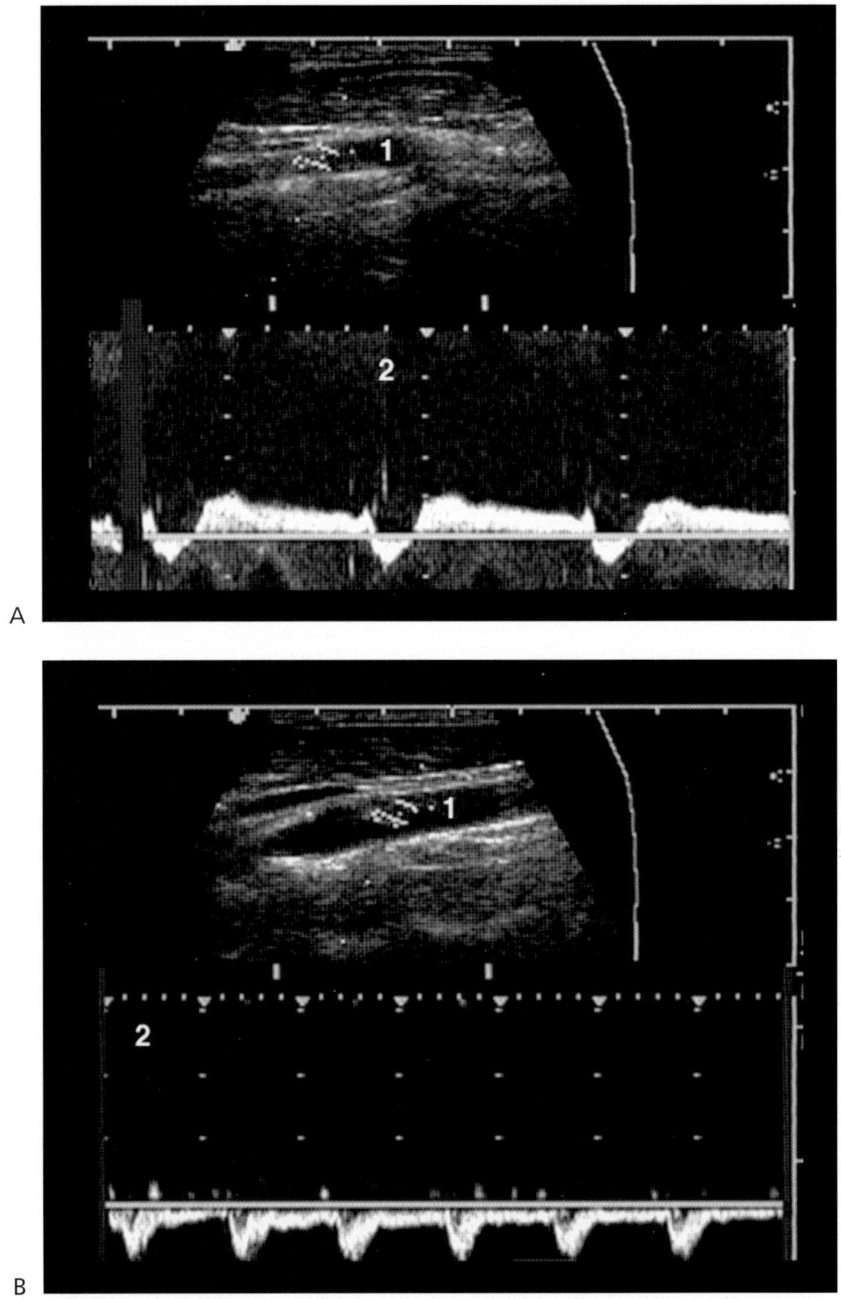

FIGURE 4.4. A: Right common carotid artery. Lateral view. Longitudinal. Gray scale. Doppler spectrum. *1*, Sample volume placed at the origin of the right common carotid artery; *2*, Doppler spectrum shows abnormal blood flow in the right common carotid artery with diminished velocity and absence of systolic velocity peaks. There is periodic reversal of blood flow direction. **B:** Right common carotid artery. Lateral view. Longitudinal. Gray scale. Doppler spectrum. Cuff test. *1*, Sample volume placed at the origin of the right common carotid artery; *2*, Doppler spectrum shows total reverse flow in the right common carotid artery after cuff release.

Diagnosis: Occlusion of the brachiocephalic artery. Stenosis or occlusions of the arteries of the upper limb are considered to be relatively rare compared with the lower limb. The most common site of arterial stenosis affecting the upper extremity is the origin of the left subclavian artery. This is a site not generally visualized directly during duplex scanning and the evidence of stenosis must be sought indirectly by the hemodynamic changes. On the right side, stenosis is less common and may affect the subclavian artery as well as the brachiocephalic artery. When the latter is stenotic or occluded, the hemodynamic changes can affect the carotid artery, as well as the subclavian and vertebral arteries. Hemodynamic alterations of the vertebral artery usually precede changes in the carotid system. The most common finding in the carotid artery is alternating blood flow direction or simply a decrease in systolic blood flow velocity. A total reversal of blood flow direction appears after the upper arm compression test (4).

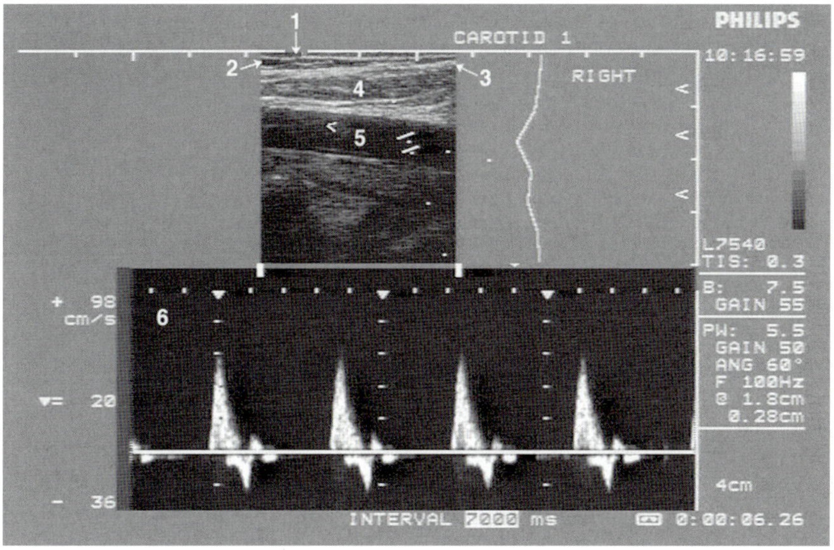

FIGURE 4.5. Right common carotid artery. Lateral view. Longitudinal. Gray scale. Doppler spectral display. *1*, Skin and superficial cervical fascia; *2*, platysma; *3*, deep cervical fascia; *4*, sternocleidomastoid muscle; *5*, right common carotid artery; *6*, Doppler spectrum placed in the proximal right common carotid artery ipsilateral to subtotal occlusion of the right internal carotid artery.

Diagnosis: Subtotal occlusion of the right internal carotid artery. A high-grade carotid artery stenosis may cause a decrease in peak systolic velocity rather than an increase. The Doppler waveform shows a high-resistance pattern in the common carotid artery ipsilateral to the subtotal occlusion of the internal carotid artery, with low peak systolic Doppler shift and essentially no diastolic flow, suggesting high resistance distally (5).

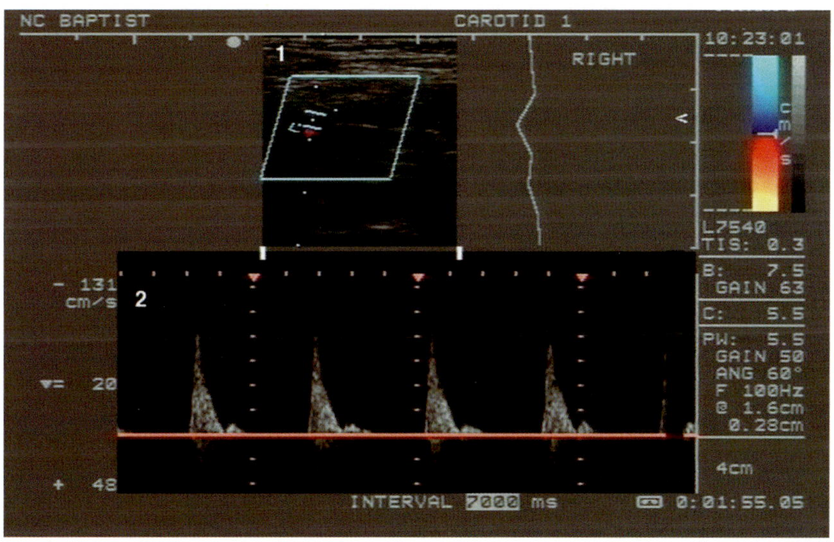

FIGURE 4.6. Right internal carotid artery. Lateral view. Longitudinal. Gray scale. Doppler spectral display. *1*, Sample volume placed at proximal right internal carotid artery; *2*, Doppler waveform proximal to the high-grade stenosis.

Diagnosis: Subtotal occlusion of the right internal carotid artery. The stenosis reaches such a level of severity that volume flow decreases below critical value and the velocities measured at the stenosis decrease. These Doppler waveforms were sampled in the internal carotid artery at a point proximal to a high-grade stenosis and show still mostly antegrade flow with decrease in diastolic flow (5).

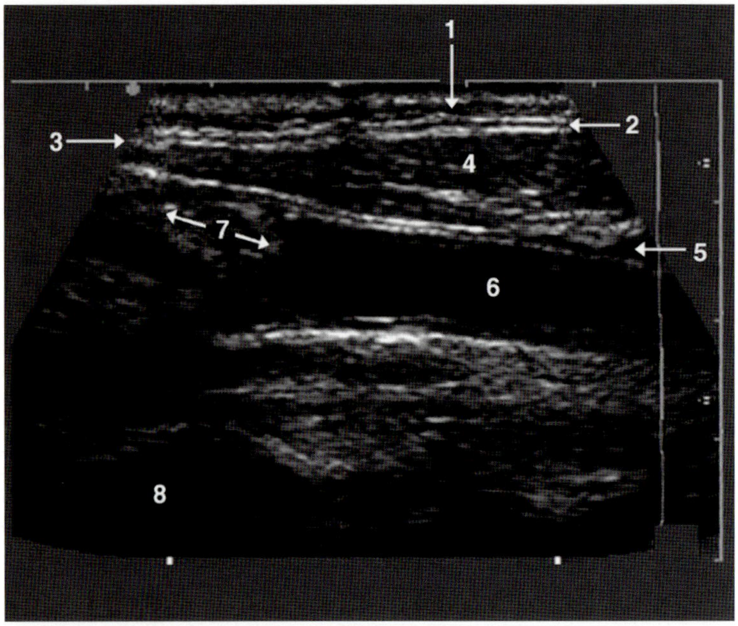

A

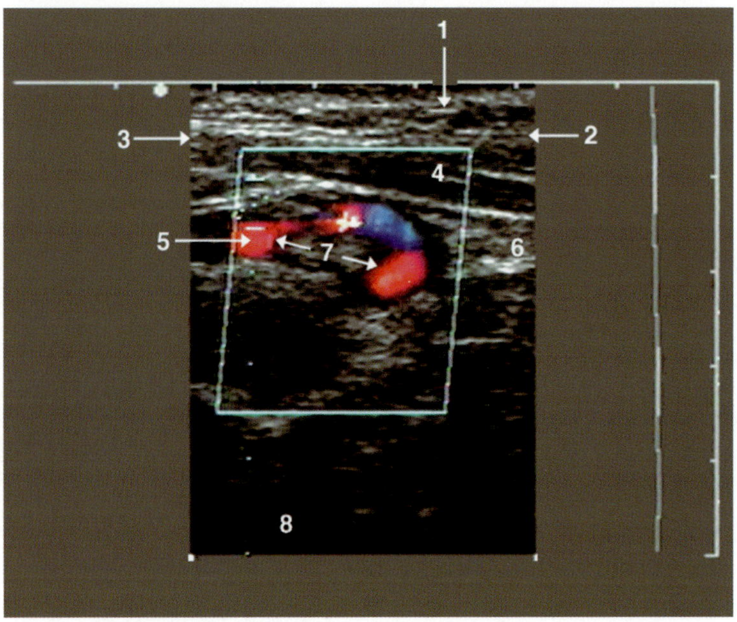

B

FIGURE 4.7. A: Bifurcation of the left common carotid artery. Lateral view. Longitudinal. Gray scale. *1*, Skin and superficial cervical fascia; *2*, platysma; *3*, deep cervical fascia; *4*, sternocleidomastoid muscle; *5*, internal jugular vein; *6*, left common carotid artery; *7*, thrombus in the lumen of the left internal carotid artery; *8*, acoustic shadowing due to the transverse process of the vertebra. **B:** Bifurcation of the left common carotid artery. Lateral view. Longitudinal. Color. *1*, Skin and superficial cervical fascia; *2*, platysma; *3*, deep cervical fascia; *4*, sternocleidomastoid muscle; *5*, flow passing around the thrombus in the left internal carotid artery; *6*, left common carotid artery; *7*, thrombus in the lumen of the left internal carotid artery; *8*, acoustic shadowing resulting from the transverse process of the vertebra.

Diagnosis: Thrombus in the lumen of the internal carotid artery. Partially thrombosed segments of the artery have echogenic material filling the lumen that move back and forth during the cardiac cycle with evidence of flow passing around the thrombus. The criteria for grading or "aging" an acute thrombus are: (a) the thrombus may be focal in nature with patent segments above and below, and it may be slightly, but not completely, compressible under the transducer; (b) the thrombus generally has a smooth surface and a "soft" homogeneous appearance. The ultrasonic tissue characterization, based on parameters obtained from the power spectrum of backscattered ultrasound signals, shows a high sensitivity, specificity, and accuracy in the correct classification of carotid plaque thrombus (6).

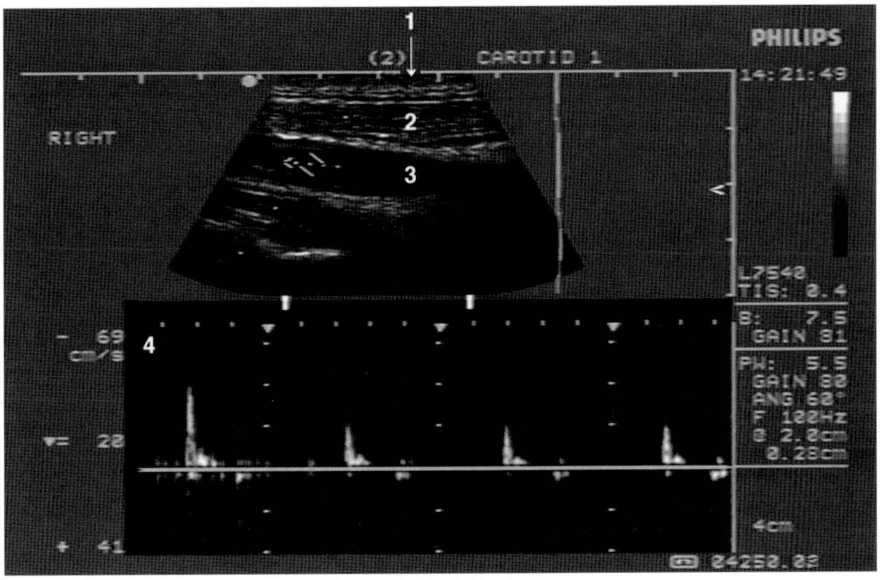

FIGURE 4.8. Right internal carotid artery. Lateral view. Longitudinal. Gray scale. Doppler spectral display. *1*, Skin and superficial cervical fascia; *2*, sternocleidomastoid muscle; *3*, right internal carotid artery; *4*, Doppler spectrum of the right internal carotid artery proximal to the occlusion with a stump sign.

Diagnosis: Internal carotid artery occlusion, stump sign. The Doppler waveform sampled in the internal carotid artery at a site proximal to a total occlusion shows a back-and-forth pattern that suggests that the blood enters in a short segment of the internal carotid artery, which is still patent, and causes distention of the walls as a result of an increased blood volume; the blood leaves this closed system when the systemic pressure decreases during diastole. This is called the stump sign (7).

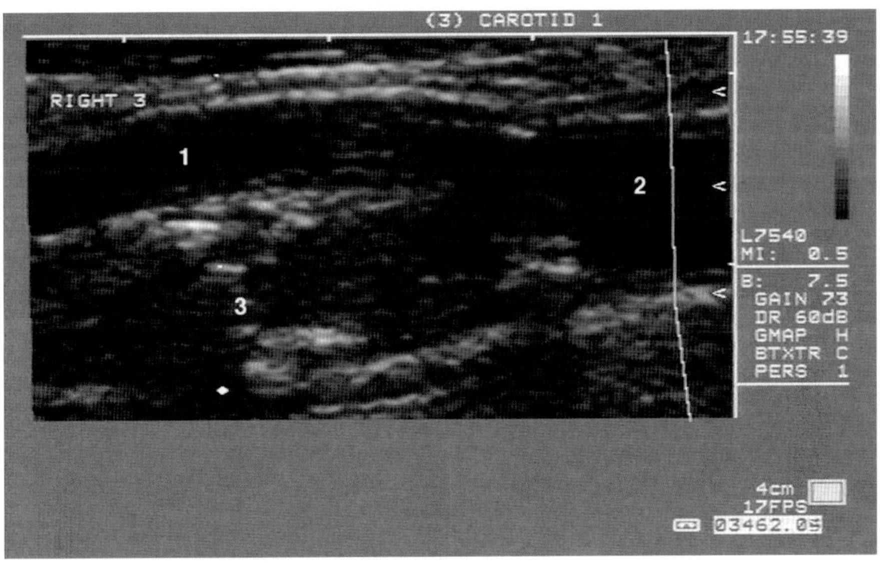

FIGURE 4.9. Right internal, external, and common carotid arteries. Posterolateral view. Longitudinal. Gray scale. *1*, Right external carotid artery; *2*, right distal common carotid artery; *3*, echogenic material fills the lumen of the right internal carotid artery.

Diagnosis: Internal carotid artery occlusion. A large amount of echogenic material fills the lumen of the internal carotid artery. To determine the appropriate diagnosis, it is necessary to identify the absence of flow in the internal carotid artery and to differentiate it from a critical stenosis with trickle flow called a "string sign" (8).

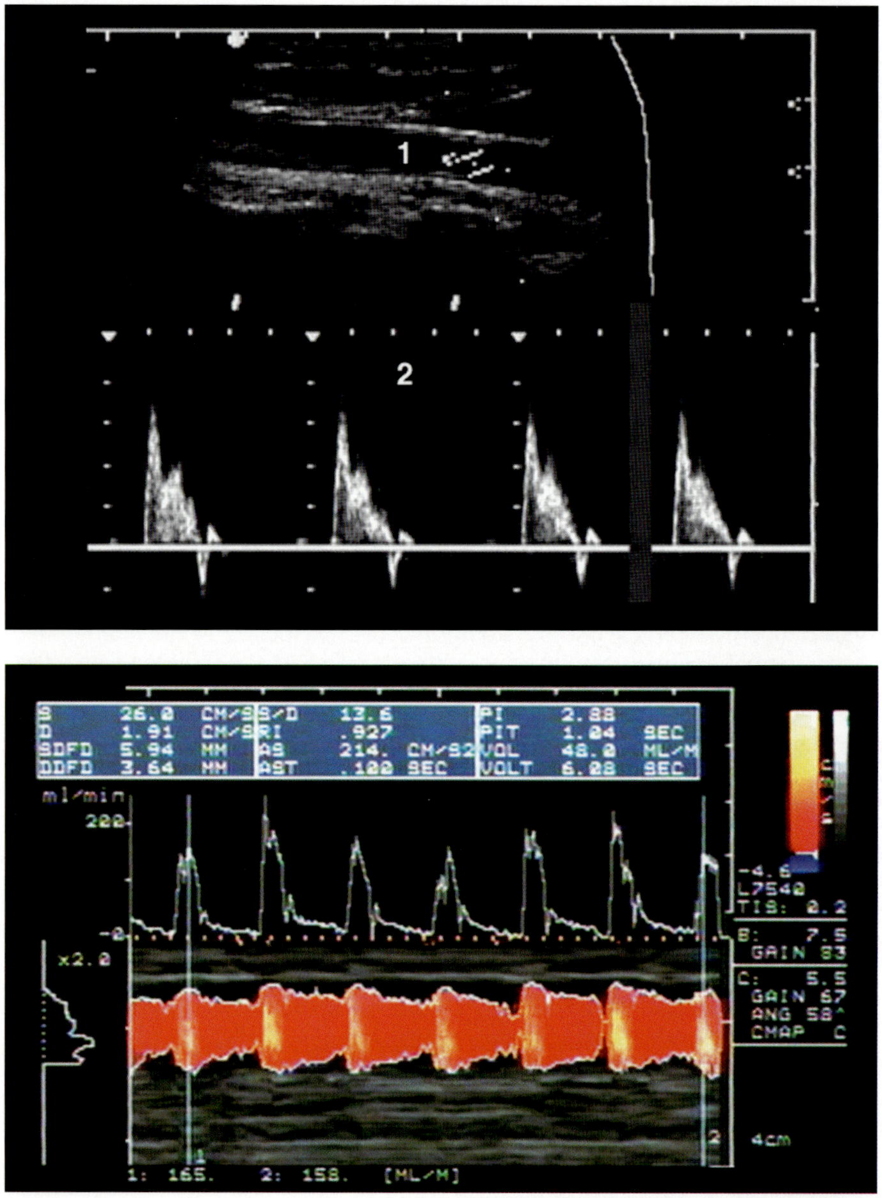

FIGURE 4.10. A: Right internal carotid artery. Lateral view. Longitudinal. Gray scale. Doppler spectrum. *1*, Sample volume placed at the origin of the right internal carotid artery; *2*, Doppler spectrum shows a high resistance flow pattern. **B:** Ultrasonic quantification of blood flow volume. M-mode display of the right common carotid artery.

Diagnosis: Occlusion of the right internal carotid artery. The clinical applications of volume flow rate measurements in stroke and cerebrovascular disease can be useful. The normal values of blood flow in the common carotid artery are 380 to 520 ml/min. Benetos and colleagues have reported a decreased volume flow rate in the ipsilateral common carotid artery, depending on the degree of internal carotid artery stenosis. Some authors have studied the effect of stenosis both ipsilaterally and contralaterally to evaluate collateral flow effects. Volume flow rate in the ipsilateral common carotid artery, proximal to greater than 90% stenosis, was about half of the normal values. In view **(B)**, the volume flow rate was 48 ml/min. Volume flow rate is the final product of many other factors and may be one of the most clinically important parameters for understanding cerebral hemodynamics and to know the risk for specific patients (9).

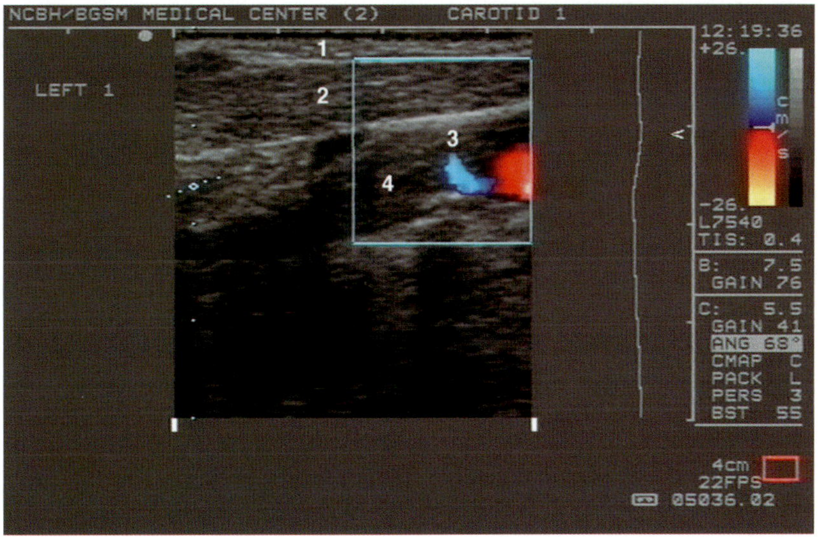

FIGURE 4.11. Left internal carotid artery. Anteroposterior view. Longitudinal. Color. *1*, Skin and superficial cervical fascia; *2*, sternocleidomastoid muscle; *3*, reversed flow at level of the occlusion of the left internal carotid artery (*blue*); *4*, echogenic material filling the lumen of the left internal carotid artery.

Diagnosis: Internal carotid artery occlusion. This color flow map shows loss of color flow signals at the site of a total occlusion. Color flow and power Doppler imaging have made specific contributions to the diagnostic capabilities of Doppler sonography, and recent data suggest that it may improve diagnostic accuracy in detecting and distinguishing total from subtotal artery occlusions (10).

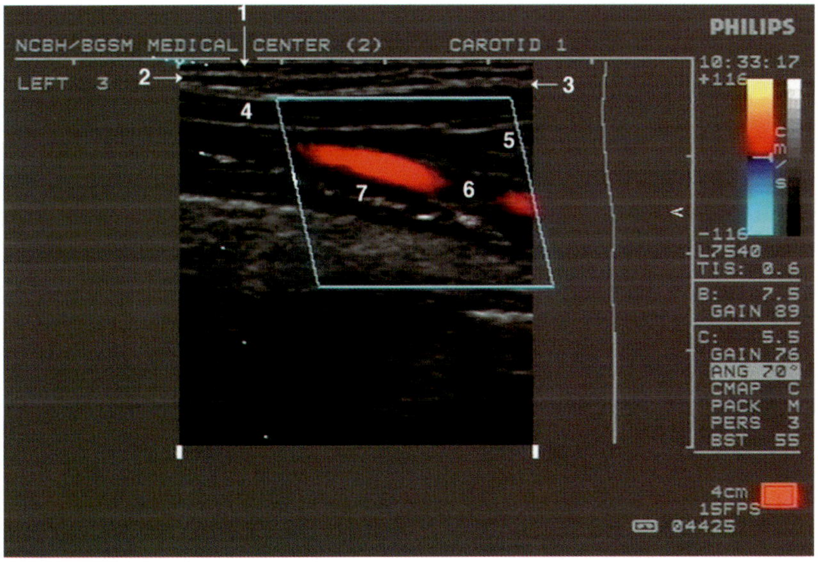

FIGURE 4.12. Left common carotid artery. Posterolateral view. Longitudinal. Color. *1*, Skin and superficial cervical fascia; *2*, platysma; *3*, deep cervical fascia; *4*, sternocleidomastoid muscle; *5*, left internal jugular vein; *6*, color flow imaging indicates antegrade flow in the residual lumen of the left common carotid artery; *7*, echogenic material filling partially the lumen of the left common carotid artery.

Diagnosis: Subtotal occlusion of the common carotid artery. Some authors have studied the efficacy of the carotid duplex ultrasound to diagnose common carotid artery occlusion (CCAO) and to define the clinical features of CCAO. The main clinical presentation is stroke, with the most common vascular risk factors being hypertension and heart disease. Duplex sonography, particularly with color-coded flow imaging, provides an accurate examination to define the patency of the residual lumen in the case of subtotal occlusion of the common carotid artery as well as the patency of the arteries distal to the carotid bifurcation in the case of CCAO (11).

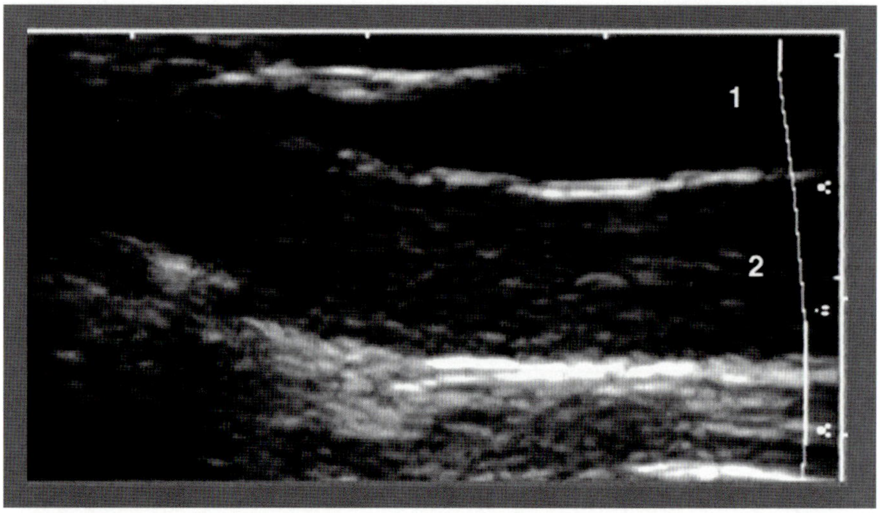

A

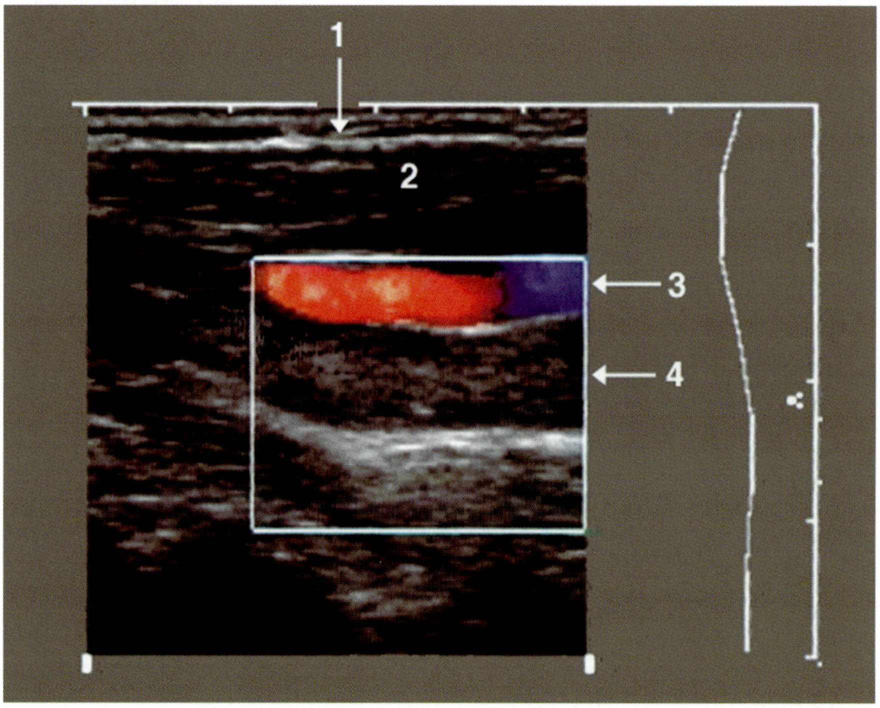

B

FIGURE 4.13. A: Right common carotid artery. Lateral view. Longitudinal. Gray scale. *1*, Right internal jugular vein; *2*, right common carotid artery. **B:** Right common carotid artery. Lateral view. Color. *1*, Skin and superficial cervical fascia; *2*, sternocleidomastoid muscle; *3*, color in the right internal jugular vein; *4*, lumen of the right common carotid artery filled with echogenic material.

Diagnosis: Common carotid occlusion. Arterial occlusion can be diagnosed with duplex imaging if the following are observed: (a) absence of arterial pulsations; (b) lumen filled with echogenic material, (c) subnormal vessel size in case of chronic occlusion, and (d) absence of flow with color duplex or Doppler signals. A false-positive diagnosis of occlusion may be made when the artery is obscured by acoustic shadowing. The flow at the internal jugular vein is seen toward and away because the ultrasound beams are focused and not cylindrical in shape, and the beam axis intersects the jugular vein at close to 90 degrees (12).

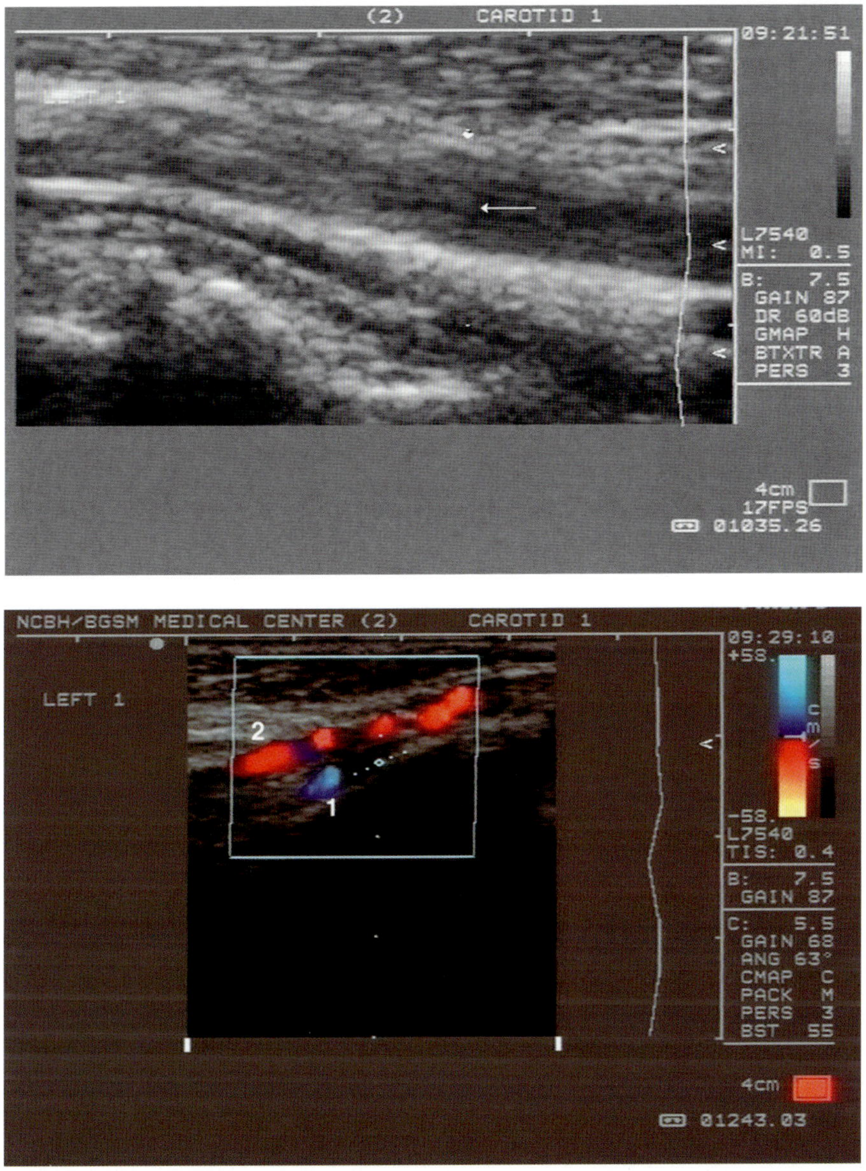

A

B

FIGURE 4.14. A: Left common carotid artery. Lateral view. Longitudinal. Gray scale. Lumen filled with echogenic material (*arrowhead*). **B**: Bifurcation of the left common carotid artery. Anteroposterior view. *1*, Retrograde flow *(blue)* in the external carotid artery; *2*, antegrade flow *(red)* in the internal carotid artery.

Diagnosis: Common carotid artery occlusion with internalization of the external carotid artery with collateral flow. The external carotid artery supplies the face and the cranium. The role of the external carotid artery as collateral to the internal carotid artery is important in pathologic situations such as common carotid artery occlusion. Occlusion of the common carotid artery is not necessarily associated with thrombosis of the ipsilateral internal and external carotid arteries. The collateral circulation through the latter may preserve the patency of the internal carotid via retrograde perfusion through the bulb. Color-coded Doppler sonography provides a correct diagnosis of the internal carotid patency in these patients with common carotid artery occlusion (13).

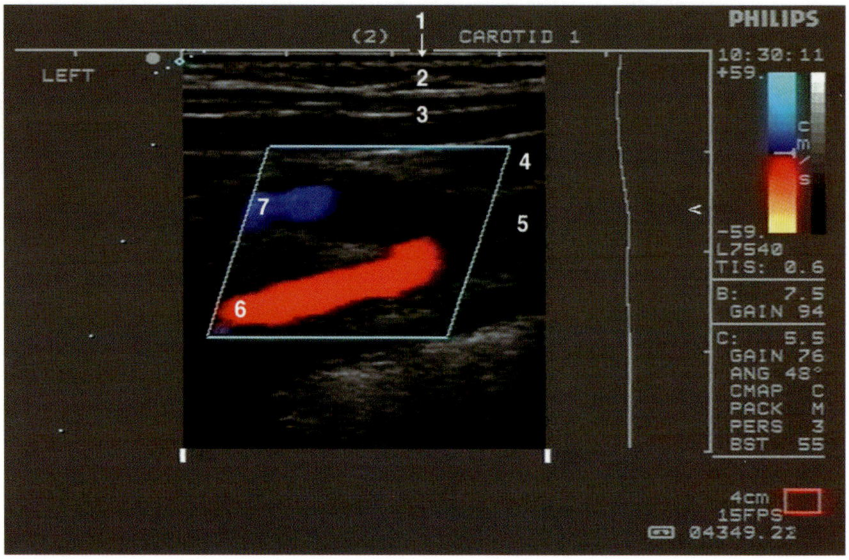

FIGURE 4.15. Bifurcation of the left common carotid artery. Lateral view. Longitudinal. Color. *1,* Skin and superficial cervical fascia; *2,* platysma; *3,* sternocleidomastoid muscle; *4,* left internal jugular vein; *5,* left common carotid artery; *6,* antegrade flow *(red)* in the left external carotid artery; *7,* retrograde flow *(blue)* in the left internal carotid artery.

Diagnosis: Subtotal occlusion of the common carotid artery with carotid steal and collateral flow. A similar altered flow that appears in the vertebral artery in the case of progression of subclavian arterial stenosis has been described in the carotid arteries with stenosis of the proximal common innominate and carotid-subclavian bypass. Some authors have proposed a phenomenologic classification of innominate artery disease following the severity of hemodynamic changes in the carotid arteries. A left internal carotid steal is shown in subtotal occlusion of the ipsilateral common carotid artery (14).

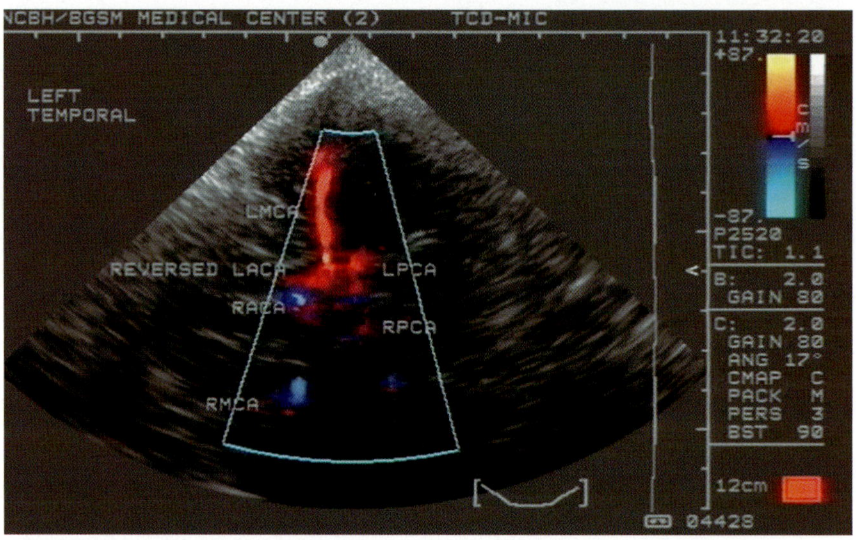

FIGURE 4.16. Transcranial color-coded duplex sonography (TCCD). Circle of Willis. Left temporal window approach. Collateral cross-flow through anterior communicating artery (*ACoA*) in the ipsilateral internal carotid artery occlusion. *LMCA,* Left middle cerebral artery; *LACA,* left anterior cerebral artery (reversed flow); *RACA,* right anterior cerebral artery; *RMCA,* right middle cerebral artery; *LPCA,* left posterior cerebral artery; *RPCA,* right posterior cerebral artery.

Diagnosis: Intracranial collateral flow with left internal carotid artery occlusion. Some studies have been performed with TCCD to establish reliable criteria for the assessment of collateral flow through the anterior (ACoA) and posterior (PCoA) communicating artery without using compression tests. In patients with adequate ultrasonic windows and internal carotid artery occlusion, the TCCD criteria for diagnosis of cross-flow through the ACoA is the detection of reversed flow in the ipsilateral anterior cerebral artery (15).

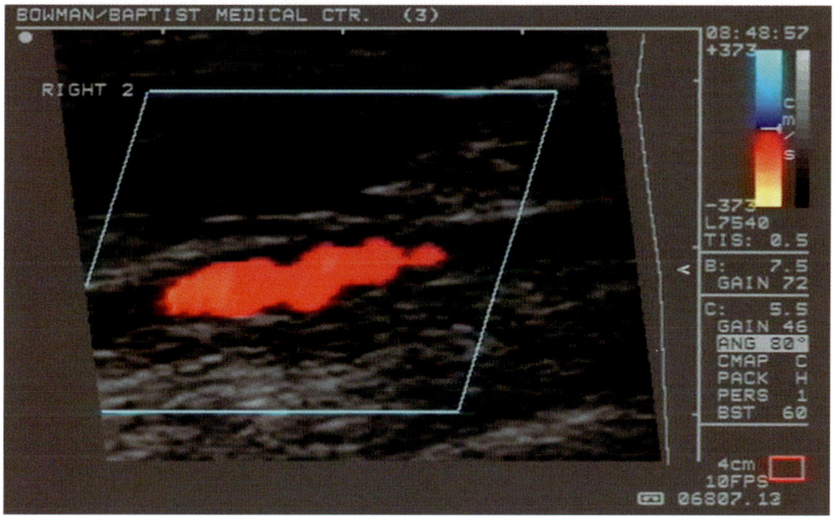

FIGURE 4.17. Right internal carotid artery. Lateral view. Color. The more distal part of the right internal carotid artery shows a spindle type of color; signal is strongly suggestive of fibromuscular dysplasia (FMD).

Diagnosis: Fibromuscular dysplasia. FMD is a vasculopathy of uncertain etiology that is histologically characterized by fibrous tissue proliferation, smooth muscle cell hyperplasia, and elastic fiber destruction alternating with segments of mural thinning. Arterial involvement is not diffuse but rather is segmental with a predisposition for long, unbranched segments of medium-sized muscular arteries. The internal carotid artery is the second most common site of FMD after the renal arteries and its characteristic beaded appearance is due to areas of medial thinning alternating with the areas of stenosis (16).

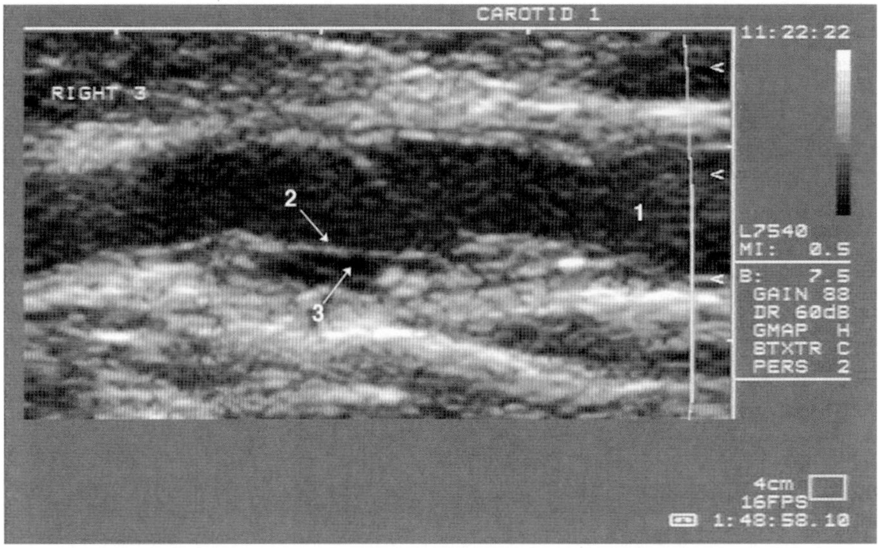

A

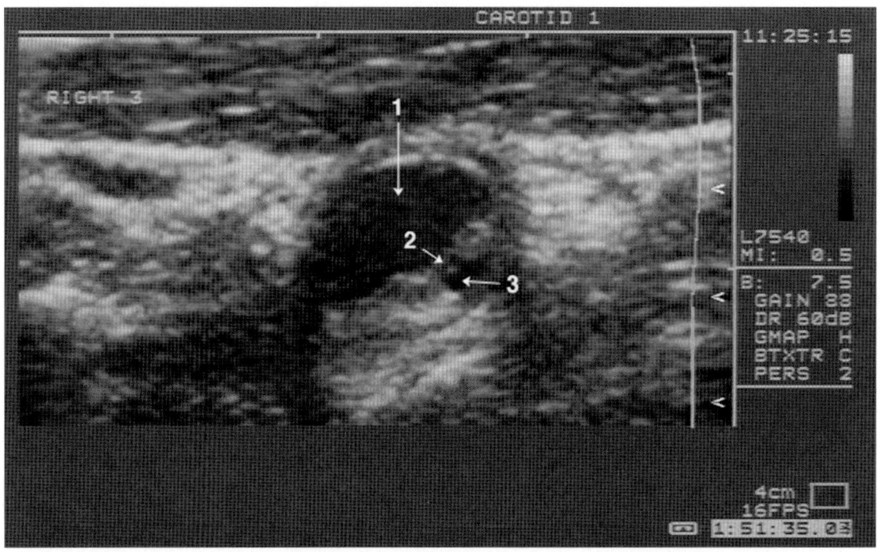

B

FIGURE 4.18. A: Right common carotid artery. Posterolateral view. Longitudinal. Gray scale. *1*, Right common carotid artery; *2*, intima dissected; *3*, false lumen. **B:** Right common carotid artery. Transverse view. Gray scale. *1*, Right common carotid artery lumen; *2*, intima dissected; *3*, false lumen.

Diagnosis: Dissection of the common carotid artery. Common carotid artery (CCA) dissection is usually found in association with a dissecting aneurysm of the aortic arch. Ultrasound studies have been reported in a limited number of cases. In contrast to internal carotid artery dissection, a typical Doppler flow pattern of CCA dissection has not yet been characterized. The B-mode evaluation of the CCA reveals a characteristic pattern of carotid dissection by clearly visualizing a vascular wall between two columns of blood. Different flow dynamics within both lumens separated by an intimal flap as well as the reentry of the false lumen are the findings in color flow imaging (17).

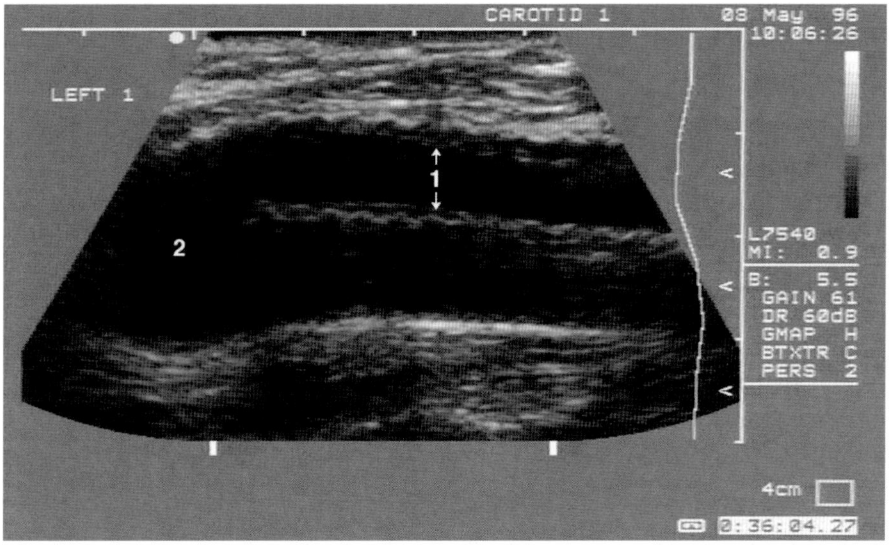

FIGURE 4.19. Left common carotid artery. Anteroposterior view. Longitudinal. Gray scale. *1*, Synthetic graft with wavelike appearance; *2*, Left common carotid wave-like artery lumen.

Diagnosis: Postsurgical findings, common carotid artery, synthetic graft. Elasticity, whether imparted by crimping or through the use of elastic materials, is a desirable but seldom achieved characteristic of a synthetic prosthesis. Any material that is elastic at implantation becomes encased in an inflexible rigid fibrous tissue sheath and loses the elasticity that might have been present (18).

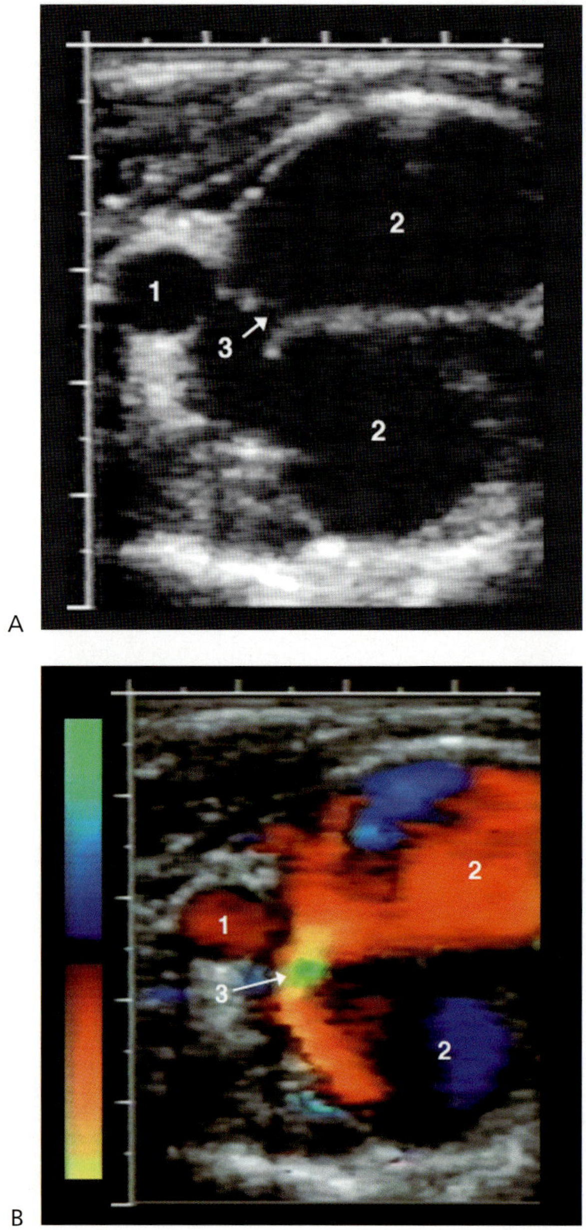

FIGURE 4.20. Left common carotid artery. Lateral view. Transverse. Gray scale **(A)** and color **(B)**. *1*, Left common carotid artery; *2*, pseudoaneurysm; *3*, neck of the pseudoaneurysm.

Diagnosis: Pseudoaneurysm of the left common carotid artery. Pseudoaneurysm is a common complication after trauma, penetrating injury, or any vascular radiologic procedure involving catheterization. Pseudoaneurysms appear sonographically as pulsatile areas anterior to the artery. Usually, a visible tract can be identified that links the mass to the artery. Color flow imaging shows the hemodynamics of these structures in detail. Pseudoaneurysms have swirling, multicolored flow patterns seen within the mass on color flow imaging. A high-velocity streamline is usually seen within the tract on color flow imaging. The outer margins of pseudoaneurysms may have thrombus surrounding a false lumen that contains a pulsatile, swirling flow. On gray-scale imaging, blood flow within the pseudoaneurysm may be swirling so slowly that blood particle motion may be seen. This must be differentiated from hematomas of the artery wall. Hematomas can be identified because there is no visible tract or pulsatile flow within them (19).

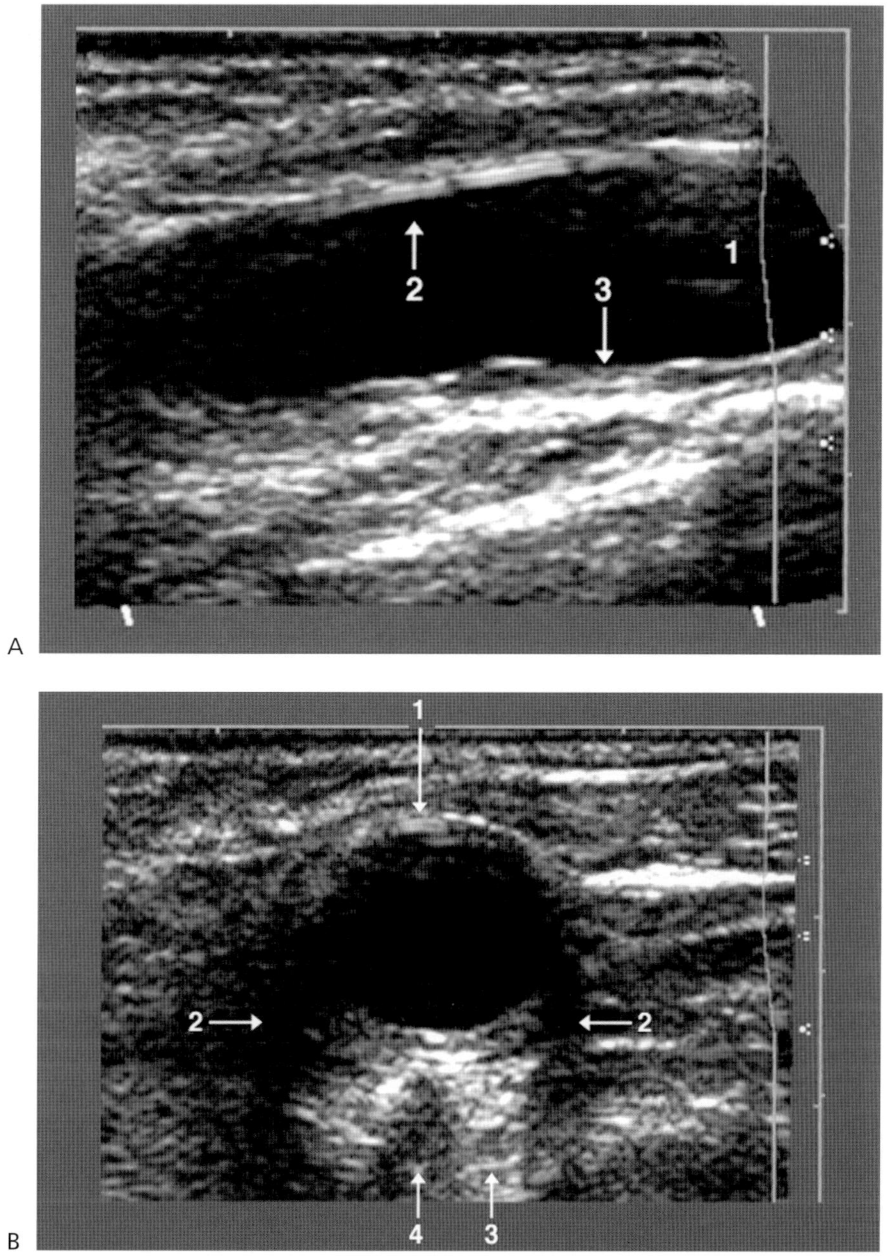

FIGURE 4.21. A: Right common carotid artery. Lateral view. Longitudinal. Gray scale. *1*, Right common carotid artery; *2*, stent wall; *3*, stent wall cover by endothelium. **B:** Right common carotid artery. Transverse view. Gray scale. *1*, Stent wall; *2*, refraction (edge) shadowing; *3*, enhancement; *4*, acoustic shadowing within the enhancement due to the stent wall.

Diagnosis: Intravascular stent in the common carotid artery. Stents are metallic coils or tubular mesh that are introduced into the body via a delivery catheter in a small or constrained diameter. An open stent wall configuration is desirable to keep thrombogenicity at a minimum and to preserve endothelium. For several months after implantation, endothelium grows to cover the stent. This is evident in the far wall of the common carotid artery of the patient shown in view **(A)**. Note the different artifacts that can appear after introduction of a metallic structure in the lumen of the vessel (20).

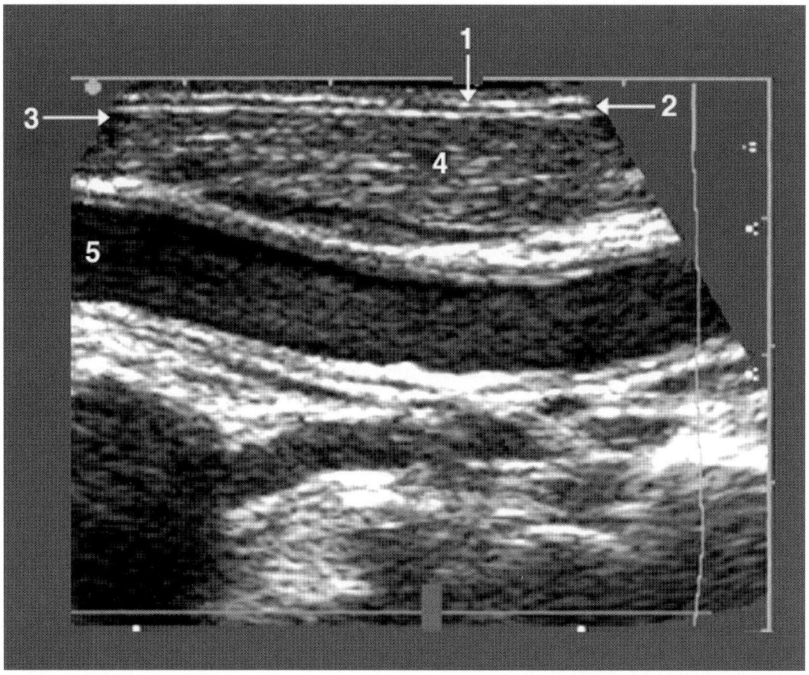

A

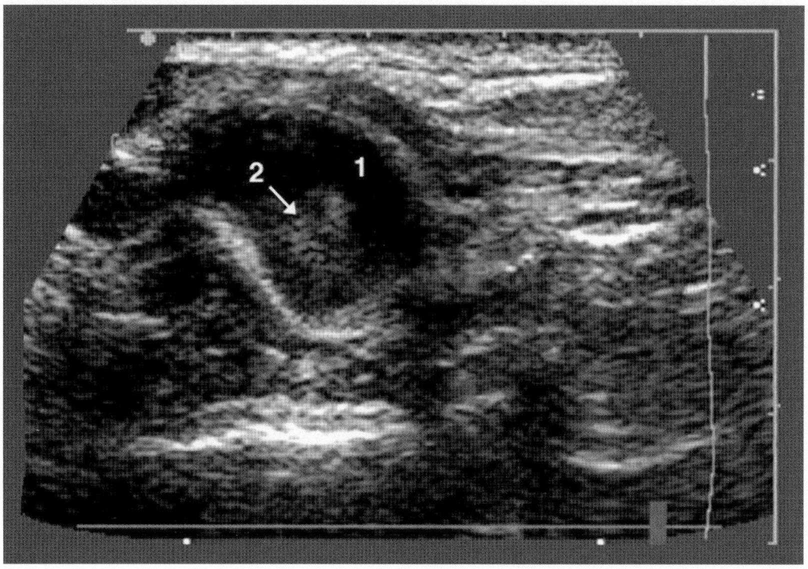

B

FIGURE 4.22. A: Right common carotid artery. Lateral view. Gray scale. Longitudinal. *1*, Skin and superficial cervical fascia; *2*, platysma; *3*, deep cervical fascia; *4*, sternocleidomastoid muscle; *5*, spontaneous echo contrast in the right common carotid artery. **B:** Right common carotid artery. Transverse view. Gray scale. *1*, Right common carotid artery; *2*, spontaneous echo contrast swirling within it.

Diagnosis: Spontaneous echo contrast in the right common carotid artery. Spontaneous echo contrast (SEC) is defined as the presence of swirling echodense shadows within the cardiac chambers or vessels. The cellular basis for SEC is generally attributed to the formation of red cell aggregates, platelet aggregates, or other factors, such as the presence of anticardiolipin antibodies, an elevated erythrocyte sedimentation rate, and increased levels of plasma fibrinogen. SEC detected within the thoracic aorta by transesophageal echocardiography has been associated with an increased risk of thromboembolism, as well as future myocardial infarction and cardiac mortality. The risk of stroke and the presence of SEC within the common carotid artery is another factor under investigation (21).

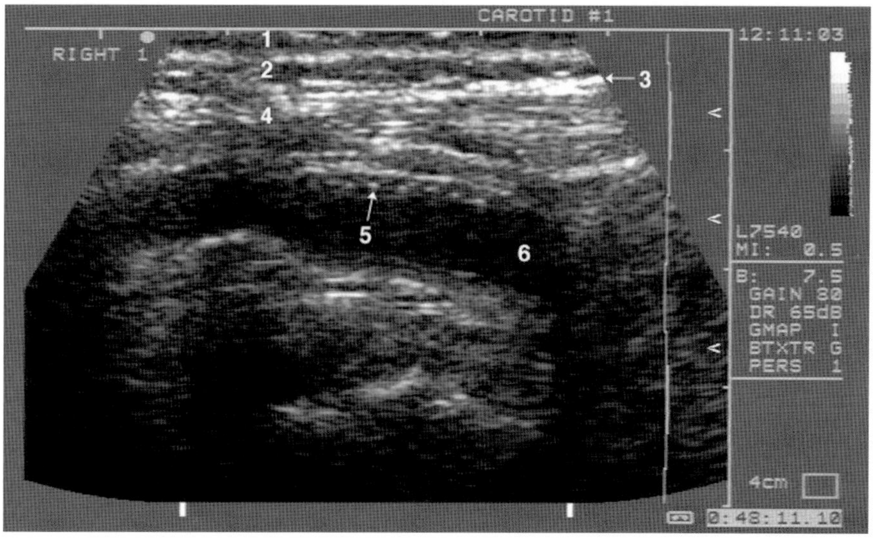

FIGURE 4.23. Right common carotid artery. Anteroposterior view. Longitudinal. Gray scale. *1*, Skin and superficial cervical fascia; *2*, platysma; *3*, deep cervical fascia; *4*, sternocleidomastoid muscle; *5*, suture line.

Diagnosis: Postsurgical findings. Suture line. There is a suture line on the near wall of the common carotid artery. There is some thickening of the near wall that is not due to recurrent or residual plaque but to serration of the artery caused by the sutures. Note the absence of a clearly defined "intimal stripe" in this endarterectomized bifurcation along the near wall (22).

PEARLS AND PITFALLS

Pearls

- Key parameters for interpreting carotid stenosis are the peak systolic and end diastolic velocities.
- The Doppler waveform sampled at a site proximal to a total occlusion of the internal carotid artery shows a back-and-forth pattern. This is the "Stump" sign.
- A diagnosis of internal carotid occlusion can be made when blood flow in the internal carotid artery is not detectable. The supporting features are the presence of the stump sign in the internal carotid artery, longitudinal pulsation of the common carotid artery, and results of ancillary testing including transcranial Doppler and ophthalmic flow.
- Visualization of a vascular wall between two columns of blood is the characteristic pattern of carotid dissection by duplex sonography.

Pitfalls

- Velocities may be "falsely" elevated in the artery contralateral to a high-grade stenosis if it is providing collateral flow.
- "Internalization" of blood flow in the external carotid artery when the internal carotid artery is occluded can lead to missing the diagnosis of internal carotid occlusion. Temporal tapping and identification of the external carotid artery branches can assist in preventing vessel misidentification.
- A false-positive diagnosis of occlusion may be made when the artery is obscured by acoustic shadowing with the absence of flow detected by color duplex or Doppler signals.
- The presence of a visible tract and pulsatile flow avoids the misdiagnosis of pseudoaneurysms as hematoma of the artery wall.

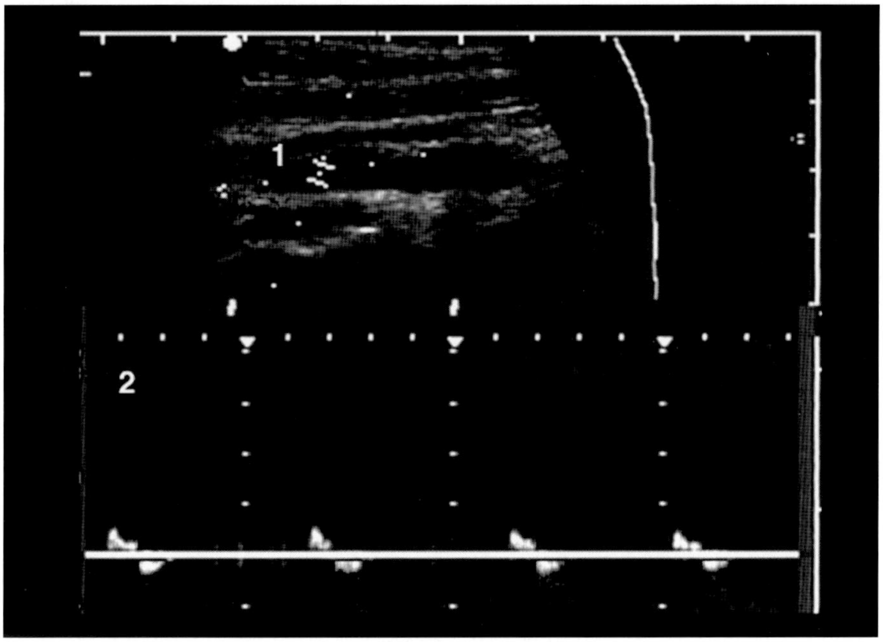

FIGURE 4.25. Left internal carotid artery. Lateral view. Longitudinal. Gray scale. Doppler spectrum. *1*, Sample placed at the origin of the left internal carotid artery; *2*, Doppler spectrum of the origin of the left internal carotid artery.

19. Which of the following statements apply to the Doppler spectrum of the origin of the left internal carotid artery shown in Figure 4.25?

  a. The spectrum shows a back-and-forth pattern Doppler waveform.
  b. This flow pattern means that the blood enters in a short, still patent segment of the artery and is pushed out during diastole.
  c. This spectrum is usually seen when there is total occlusion of the insonated artery.
  d. All of the above
  e. None of the above

20. **Diagnosis: Right internal carotid artery occlusion** (Fig. 4.26). The presence of a high-resistance Doppler waveform in the right common carotid artery, with no Doppler signal in the ipsilateral internal carotid artery and the absence of color at the same artery in transverse view, is usually associated with

a. poor cardiac output.
b. occlusion of the right internal carotid artery.
c. high-grade stenosis of the right common carotid artery.
d. All of the above
e. None of the above

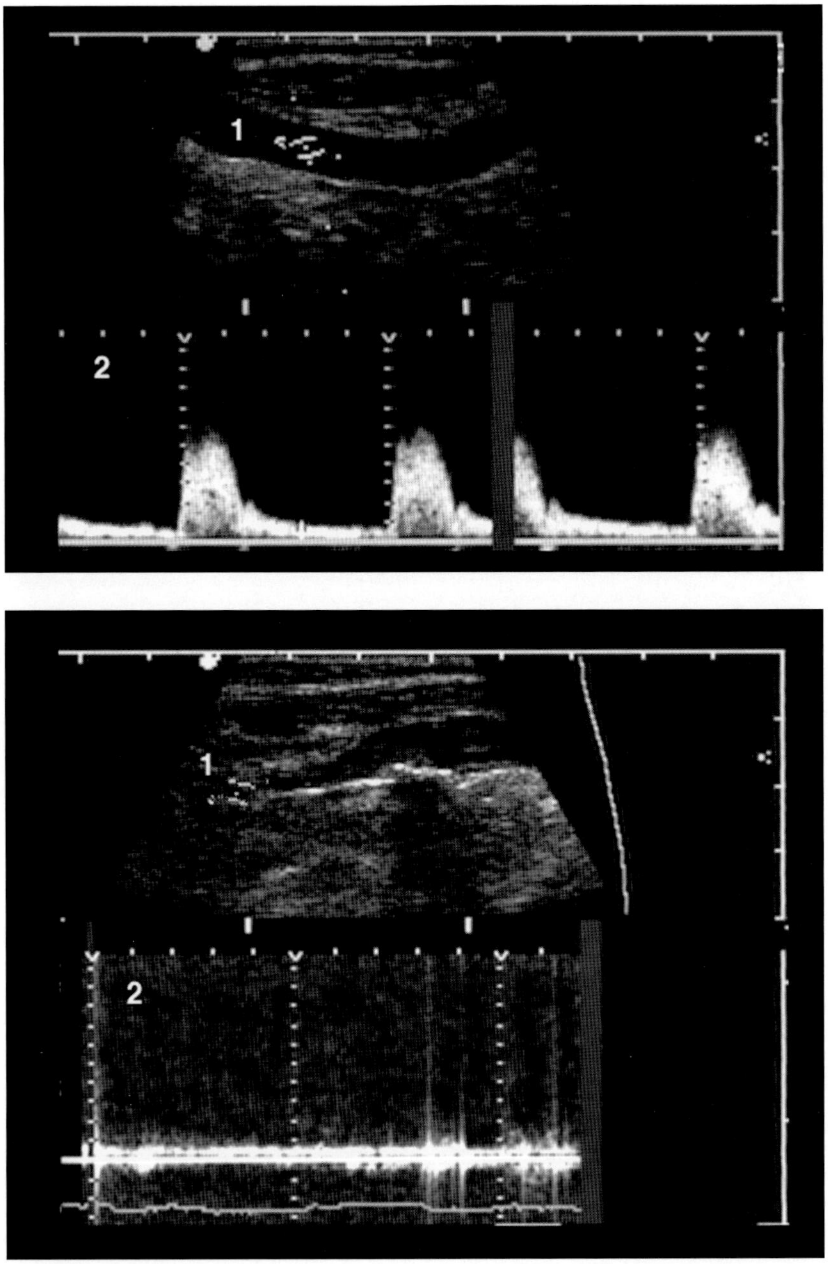

A

B

FIGURE 4.26. A: *1*, Sample volume placed in the right common carotid artery; *2*, Doppler spectrum of the right common carotid artery. **B:** Sample volume placed in the right internal carotid artery; *2*, Doppler spectrum of the right internal carotid artery.

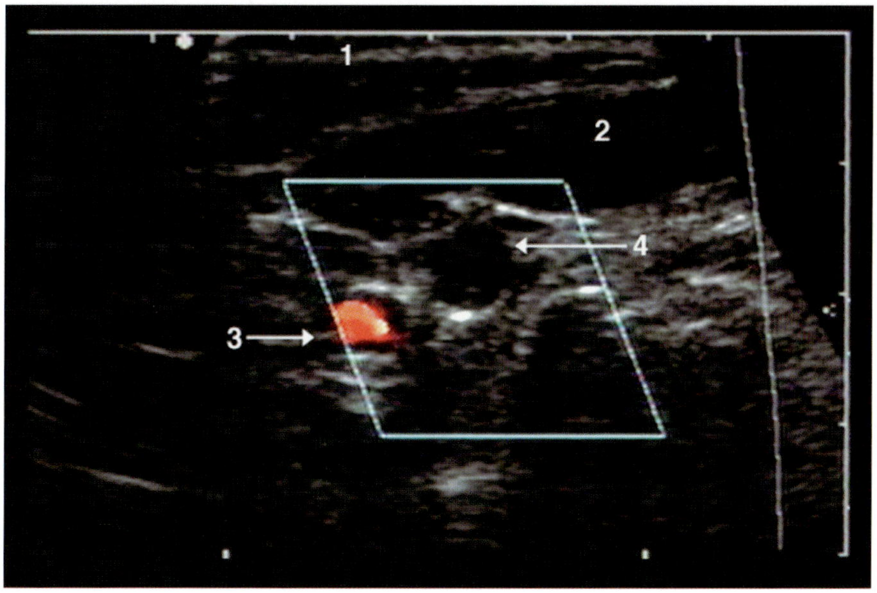

C

FIGURE 4.26. ***(continued)*** **C:** Bifurcation of the right common carotid artery. Transverse view. Gray scale. Color. *1*, Skin and superficial cervical fascia; *2*, sternocleidomastoid muscle; *3*, right external carotid artery; *4*, right internal carotid artery.

Answers: 1. a; **2.** True; **3.** d; **4.** e; **5.** e; **6.** True; **7.** e; **8.** d; **9.** False; **10.** d; **11.** a; **12.** d; **13.** e; **14.** b; **15.** True; **16.** b; **17.** a; **18.** True; **19.** d; **20.** b.

REFERENCES

1. Zwiebel W. New Doppler parameters for carotid stenosis. *Semin Ultrasound CT MR* 1997;18:66–71.
2. Päivänsalo MJ, Siniluoto TMJ, Tikkakoski TA, et al. Duplex ultrasound of the external carotid artery. *Acta Radiologica* 1996;37(1):41–45.
3. Breslau PJ, Fell F, Phillips DJ, et al. Evaluation of carotid bifurcation disease: the role of common carotid velocity waveform patterns. *Arch Surg* 1982;117:58–60.
4. Brunhoelzl C, von Reutern GM. Hemodynamic effects of innominate artery occlusive disease. Evaluation by Doppler ultrasound. *Ultrasound Med Biol* 1989;15:201–204.
5. Spencer MP, Reid JM. Quantitation of carotid stenosis with continuous-wave (c-w) Doppler ultrasound. *Stroke* 1979;10:326–330.
6. Noritomi T, Sigel B, Gahtan V, et al. In vivo detection of carotid plaque: thrombus by ultrasonic tissue characterization. *J Ultrasound Med* 1997;16(2):107–111.
7. Polak JF. Color flow imaging of the carotid arteries. In: Tegeler CH, Babikian VL, Gomez CR, eds. *Neurosonology.* Chicago: Mosby–Year Book, 1996.
8. Krebs CA, Giyanani VL, Eisenberg RL. *Ultrasound atlas of disease processes.* Norwalk, CT: Appleton & Lange, 1993.
9. Tegeler CH, Knappertz VA, Eicke BM, et al. Carotid artery volume flow rate correlates with severity of stenosis. *Radiology* 1994;193:231.
10. Hetzel A, Eckenweber B, Trummer B, et al. Color-coded duplex ultrasound in preocclusive stenosis of the internal carotid artery. *Ultraschall Med* 1993;14:240–246.
11. Chang YJ, Lin SK, Ryu SJ, et al. Common carotid artery occlusion: evaluation with duplex sonography. *Am J Neuroradiol* 1995;16:1099–1105.
12. Steinke W, Kloetzsch C, Hennerici M. Carotid artery disease assessed by color Doppler flow imaging: correlation with standard Doppler sonography and angiography. *Am J Roentgenol* 1990;154:1061–1068.
13. Trattrug S, Hubsch P, Barton P, et al. The patency of the external and internal carotid arteries in patients with occlusion of the common carotid: detection using color-coded Doppler sonography. *Rofo* 1991;154:44–48.
14. Schwend RB, Hambsch K, Baker L, et al. Carotid steal syndrome: a case study. *J Neuroimaging* 1995;5:195–197.
15. Baumgartner RW, Baumgartner I, Schroth G. Diagnostic criteria for transcranial color-coded duplex sonography evaluation of cross-flow through the circle of Willis in unilateral obstructive carotid artery disease. *J Neurol* 1996;243:516–521.
16. Schievink WI, Bjornsson J. Fibromuscular dysplasia of the internal carotid artery: a clinicopathological study. *Clin Neuropathol* 1996;15:2–6.
17. Bashour TT, Crew JP, Dean M, et al. Ultrasonic imaging of common carotid artery dissection. *J Clin Ultrasound* 1985;13:210–211.
18. Lindenauer SM. The fabric vascular prosthesis. In: Rutherford RB, ed. *Vascular surgery,* 3rd ed. Vol 1. Philadelphia: WB Saunders, 1989.
19. Hagen-Ansert SL. *Diagnostic ultrasonography,* 4th ed. Vol 1. Chicago: Mosby–Year Book, 1995.
20. Palmaz JC. Intravascular stents: experimental observations and anatomopathologic correlates. In: Maynar-Moliner M, Castañeda-Zúñiga W, Joffre F, et al, eds. *Percutaneous revascularization techniques.* Thieme, 1993.
21. Steinberg EH, Madmon L, Wesolowsky H, et al. Prognostic significance of spontaneous echo contrast in the thoracic aorta: relation with accelerated clinical progression of coronary artery disease. *J Am Coll Cardiol* 1997;30:71–75.
22. Cranley JJ, Karkow WS, Baldridge ED. *Atlas of duplex scanning. Carotid arteries.* Philadelphia: WB Saunders, 1989.

CHAPTER 5

MORPHOLOGIC ASPECTS OF THE PLAQUE

Atheromatous plaque of the carotid artery system may impair cerebral circulation by causing emboli, flow restricting stenosis, or occlusion. Research indicates that the appearance of the carotid plaque as well as surface characteristics may play an important role in the pathogenesis of brain ischemia.

Real-time B-mode ultrasonography has become a standard part of imaging of the extracranial carotid vessels and allows examination of plaque morphology.

There is ongoing research to investigate the role of B-mode and color-coded Doppler imaging in characterizing pathologic plaque morphology and in predicting high-risk patients.

It is important to scan in both transverse and sagittal planes to accurately assess the relationship of the plaque to the wall. The ultrasonographer should record the following descriptions of the plaque: location, size, composition, and surface characteristics.

The homogenous plaque usually shows low-level echogenicity and, occasionally, increased echogenicity. Heterogeneous plaque shows a complex echo pattern that contains at least one focal sonolucent area. Sonolucency may represent ulceration, intraplaque hemorrhage, thrombosis, or lipid deposition. Heterogeneous, sonolucent, and ulcerated plaques may be associated with a greater risk of stroke.

Color flow Doppler imaging superimposes a two-dimensional, color-coded, real-time Doppler image of intravascular blood flow on the gray-scale B-mode image of vessel characteristics. Advantages of adding Doppler color imaging are better delineation of vessel anatomy, detection of hypoechoic plaque, and better definition of the surface features of plaque.

PATHOLOGICAL FEATURES OF ATHEROMATOUS PLAQUE

The following cases provide sonographic images that identify the important pathologic features of atheromatous plaque.

B-Mode Evaluation of the Carotid Plaque

B-mode examination allows the evaluation of plaque echogenicity, structure and surface characteristics. Another value of an ultrasound scan in the assessment of plaque is its superiority over an arteriogram in allowing the measurement of the composition of a particular plaque. Classification is based on the echo pattern within the plaque as assessed by two criteria. The first is the echogenicity or brightness. Plaque echogenicity has been evaluated in some studies using a scale from 1 to 3, where 1 denotes strong echoes and 3 denotes low echogenicity or echolucency. The second criterion is the degree of uniformity of the echo pattern within the plaque, which is called *homogeneity,* and plaques can be judged as homogeneous or heterogeneous. The former consists of plaque that is relatively uniform in texture compared with the soft tissues surrounding the vessel wall. The latter consists of plaque that has a complex echo pattern and contains at least one well-defined focal echolucent area.

The plaque surface is described as either regular or irregular. If there is acoustic shadowing behind the brightly echogenic areas, the plaque has areas of calcium. Calcification can be present in either form of plaque and does not enter into the scheme of classification (1).

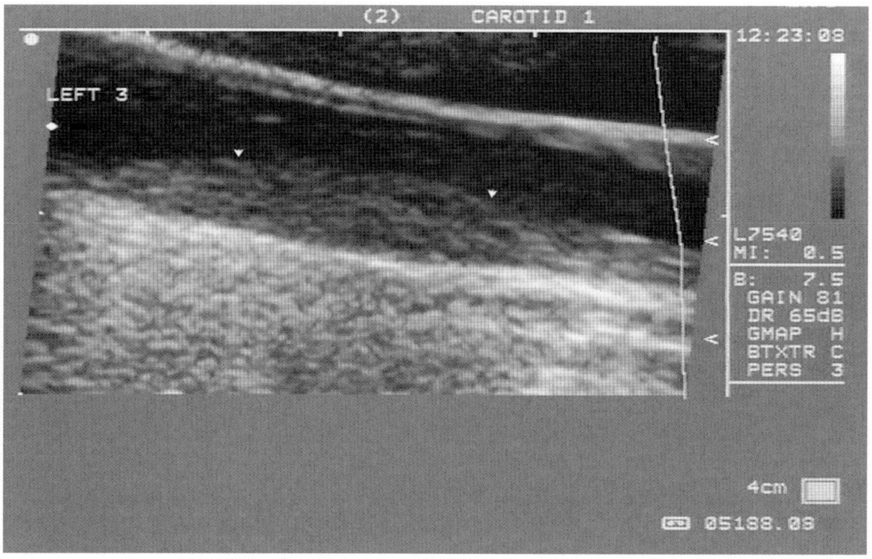

FIGURE 5.1. Left common carotid artery. Posterolateral view. Longitudinal. Gray scale. Faintly echogenic-homogeneous plaque (*arrowheads*).

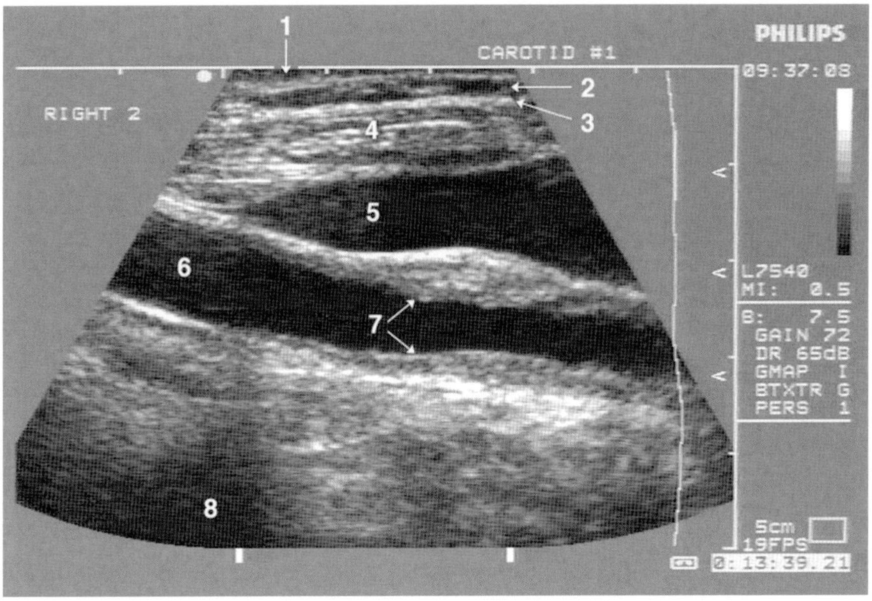

FIGURE 5.2. Right common carotid artery. Lateral view. Longitudinal. Gray scale. *1*, Skin and superficial cervical fascia; *2*, platysma; *3*, deep cervical fascia; *4*, sternocleidomastoid muscle; *5*, right internal jugular vein; *6*, right common carotid artery; *7*, brightly echogenic-homogeneous plaque; *8*, acoustic shadowing resulting from transverse process of the vertebra.

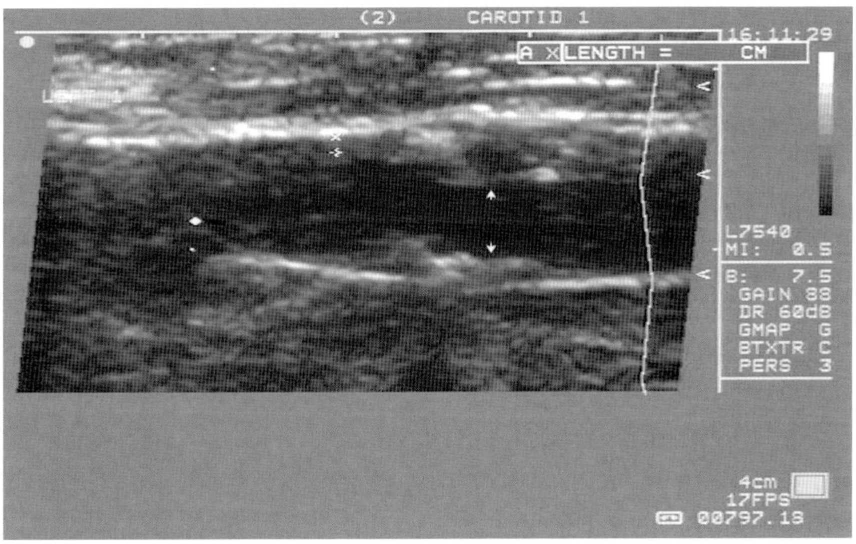

FIGURE 5.3. Left internal carotid artery. Lateral view. Longitudinal. Gray scale. Brightly echogenic-heterogeneous plaque (*arrowheads*).

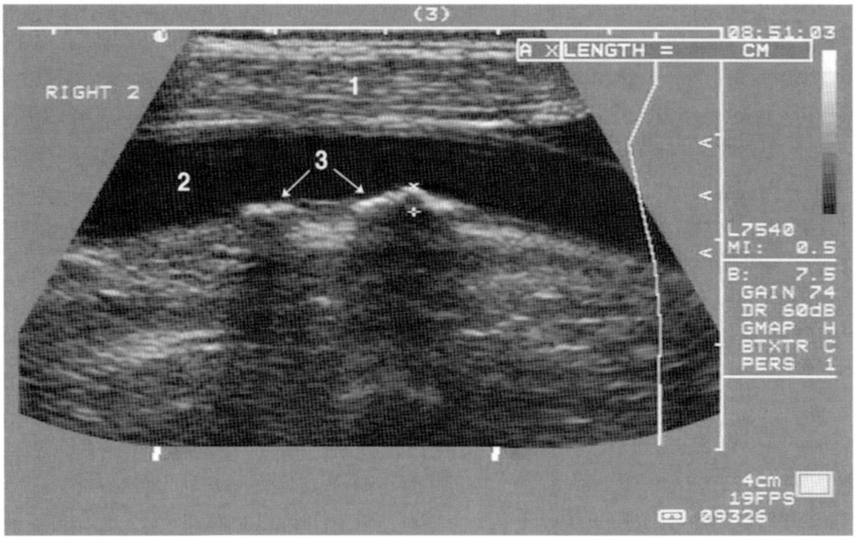

FIGURE 5.4. Right common carotid artery. Lateral view. Longitudinal. Gray scale. *1*, Sternocleidomastoid muscle; *2*, right common carotid artery; *3*, calcific plaques with acoustic shadowing.

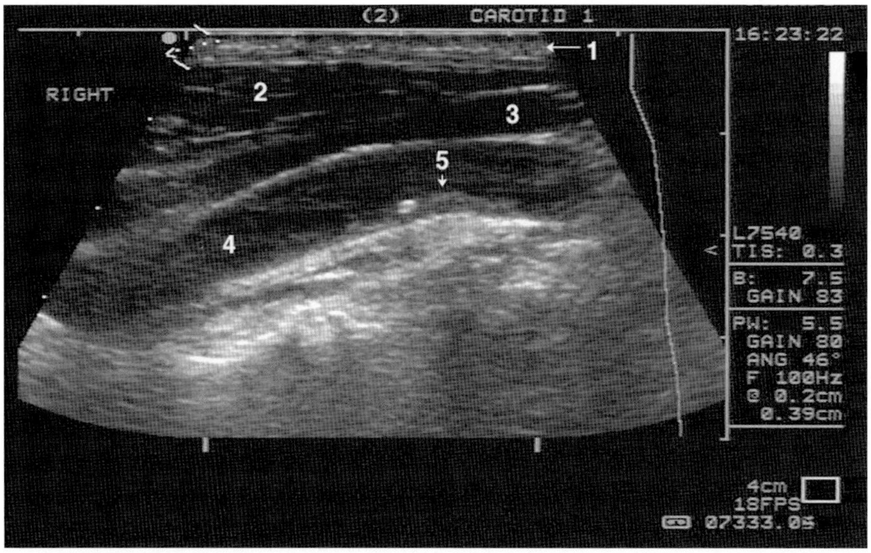

FIGURE 5.5. Homogeneous plaque in the inner wall of the right common carotid artery curvature. *1*, Skin and superficial cervical fascia; *2*, sternocleidomastoid muscle; *3*, right internal jugular vein; *4*, right common carotid artery; *5*, homogeneous plaque.

Diagnosis: Common carotid artery. Homogeneous plaque. The variation in arterial wall pressure depends on the variation in velocity with the radius of the curvature of the streamlines. The velocity increases as the radius decreases and the pressure increases with radius in a curved flow. A localized decrease in static pressure in the inner curvature produces a local suction action upon the wall. The intimal response is a local biologic change that evokes the development of atherosclerosis (2).

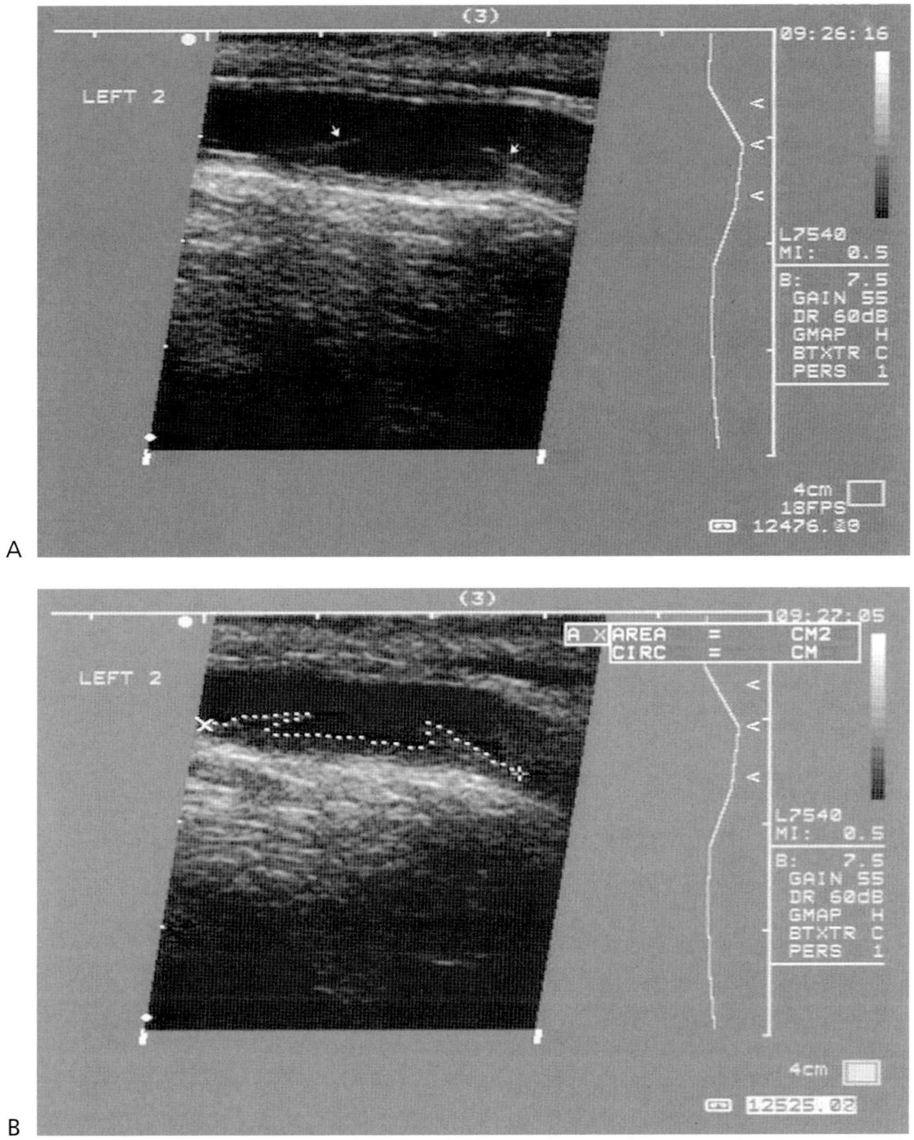

FIGURE 5.6. Left common carotid artery. Homogeneous plaque with crater (*dotted line*).

Diagnosis: Faintly echogenic plaque. Crater. The clinical importance of ulceration has been pointed out by several authors. The ability to identify ulcerations with ultrasound remains controversial. The sensitivity of ultrasound in predicting ulceration ranges from less than 30% to greater than 90% (3).

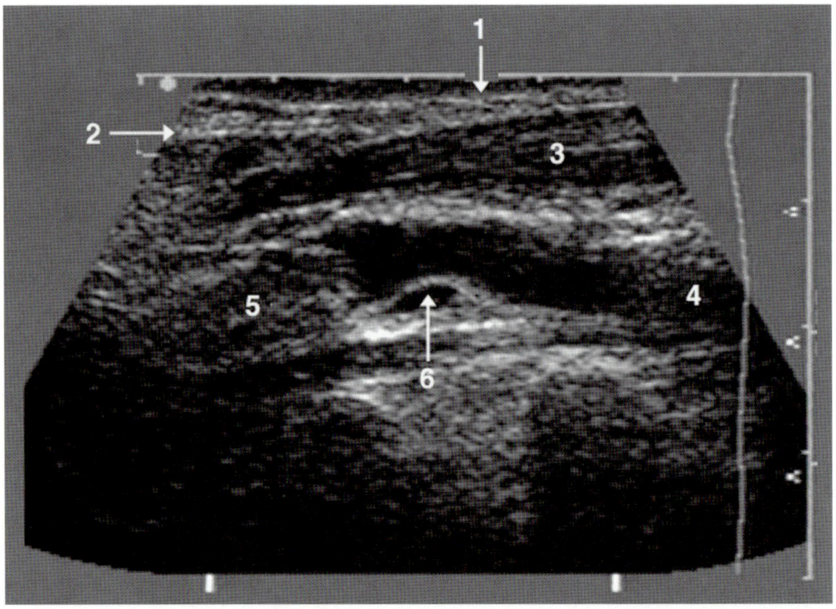

A

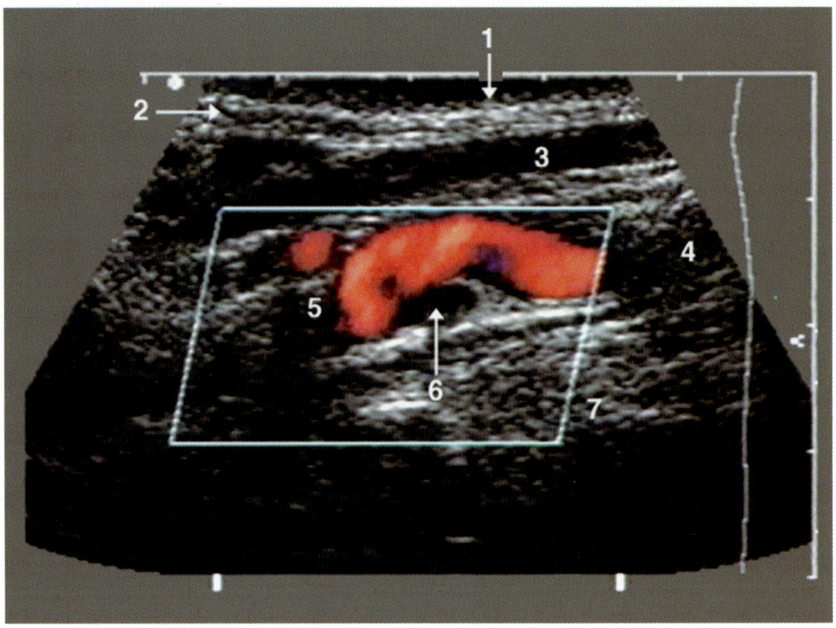

B

FIGURE 5.7. Left common and internal carotid artery. Lateral view. Longitudinal. Gray scale **(A)** and color **(B)**. *1*, Skin and superficial cervical fascia; *2*, platysma and deep cervical fascia; *3*, sternocleidomastoid muscle; *4*, left common carotid artery; *5*, left internal carotid artery; *6*, focal low-echogenicity area, which probably represents a focal intraplaque hemorrhage; *7*, color box.

Diagnosis: Heterogeneous plaque vs. intraplaque hemorrhage. Ultrasonography is a unique method to assess plaque composition. Plaque characteristics may have prognostic value and may be useful for the selection of medical or surgical therapy. Lack of homogeneity in the plaque composition seems to be the most important feature in defining the risk of embolization or rapid plaque progression. It is believed that either form of nonhomogeneity increases the risk for stroke. Focal areas of low echogenicity may be produced either by lipid or thrombus deposits. Some authors have found sonography to be 95% sensitive for detection of intraplaque hemorrhage but only 77% specific. Color flow imaging might be useful to distinguish between intraplaque hemorrhage and ulcerated carotid plaque. Color flow imaging in this case does not show any zone of flow reversal in the sonolucent area, which could be an intraplaque hemorrhage (4).

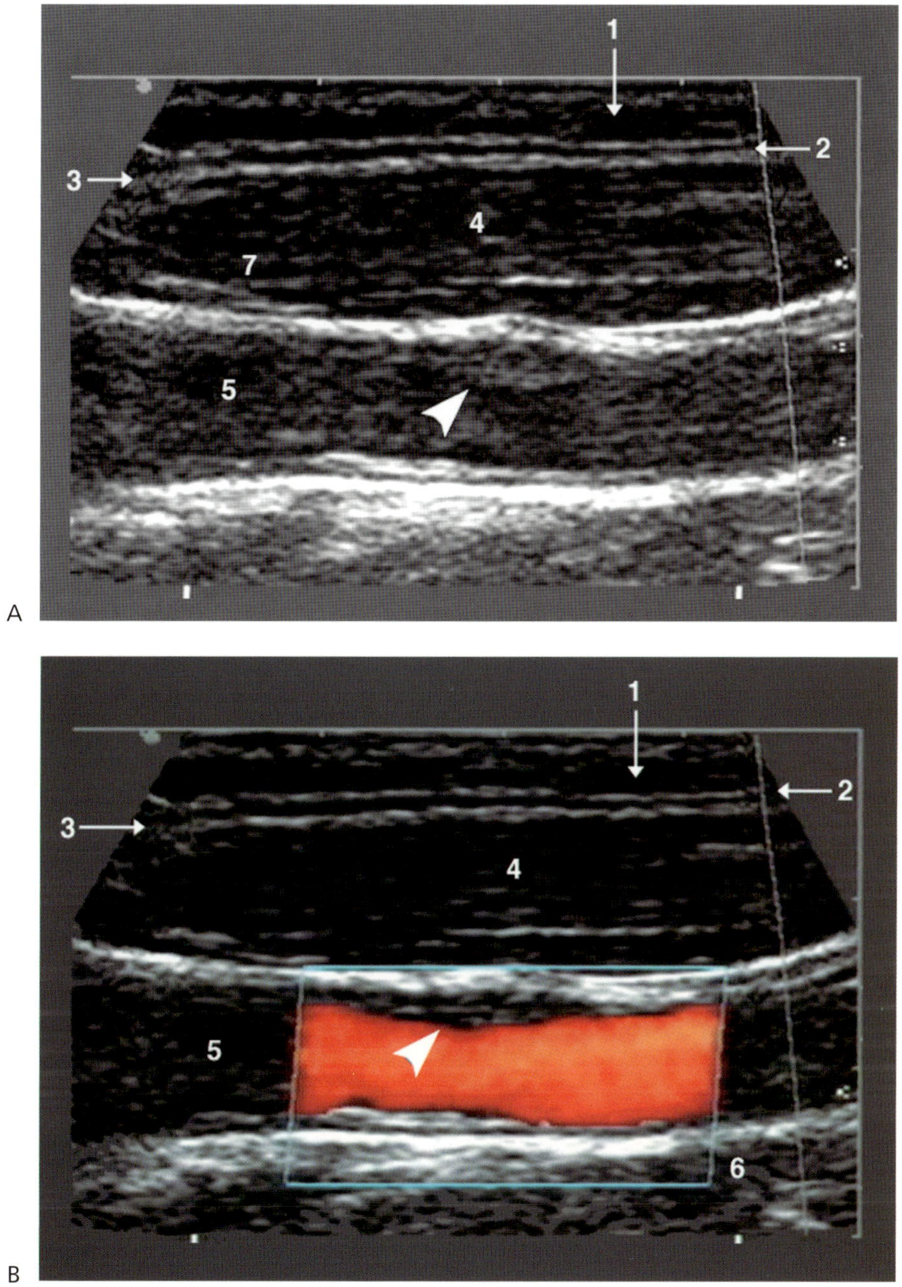

FIGURE 5.8. A: Left common carotid artery. Lateral view. Longitudinal. Gray scale. *1*, Skin and superficial cervical fascia; *2*, platysma; *3*, deep cervical fascia; *4*, sternocleidomastoid muscle; *5*, left common carotid artery; hypoechoic plaque (*arrowhead*). **B:** Left common carotid artery. Lateral view. Longitudinal. Color. *1*, Skin and superficial cervical fascia; *2*, platysma; *3*, deep cervical fascia; *4*, sternocleidomastoid muscle; *5*, left common carotid artery; *6*, color box; hypoechoic plaque (*arrowhead*).

Diagnosis: Hypoechoic plaque. By means of color flow imaging, there is excellent delineation of vessel wall irregularities. It is very useful in cases of low-echodensity plaques or thrombus formation, which might go undetected on conventional gray-scale imaging. The outline of the hypoechoic plaque is clearly shown with color-coded Doppler sonography. High-resolution sonography assisted by color flow mapping promises a higher accuracy in plaque structure analysis, as well as in measurement of plaque size, and has become part of the standard clinical examination (5).

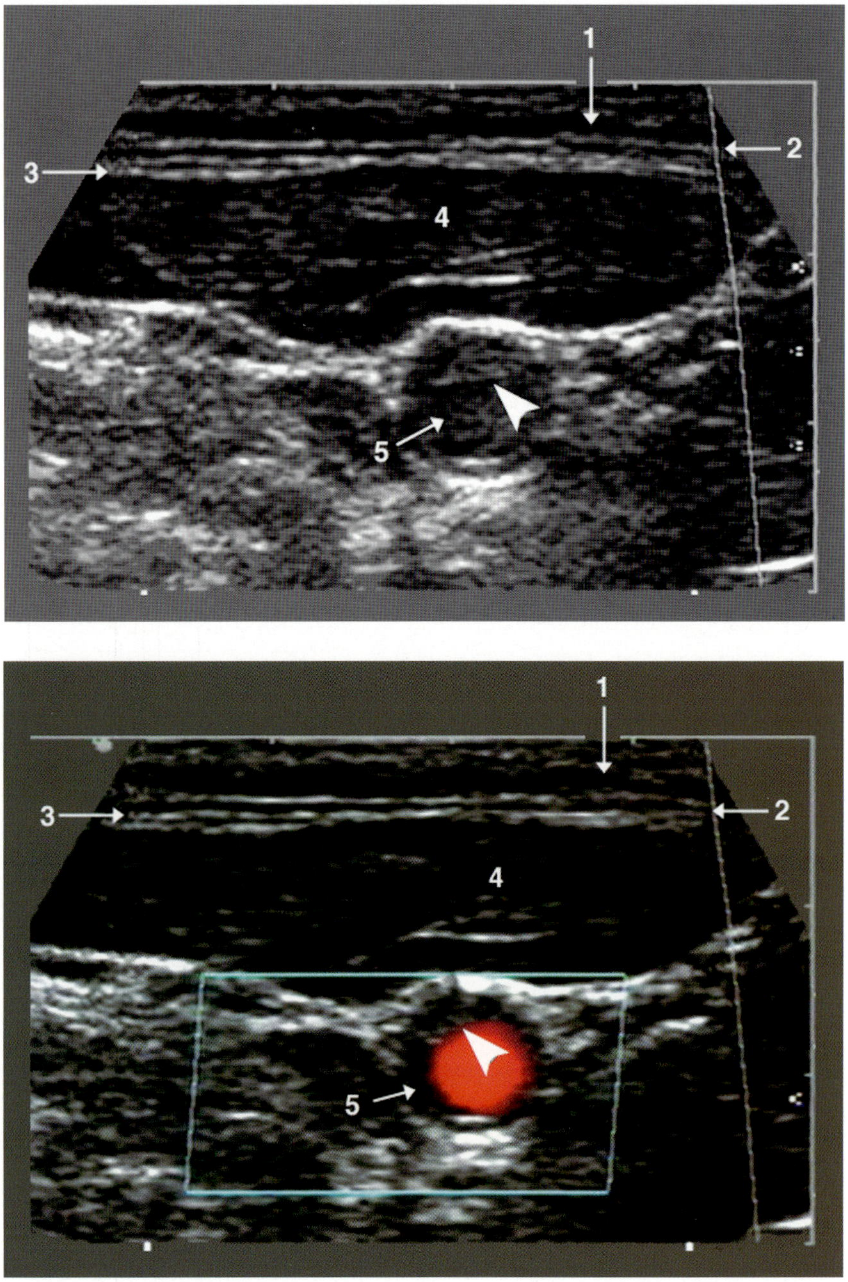

A

B

FIGURE 5.9. Left common carotid artery. Transverse view. Gray scale **(A)** and color **(B)**. *1*, Skin and superficial cervical fascia; *2*, platysma; *3*, deep cervical fascia; *4*, sternocleidomastoid muscle; *5*, left common carotid artery; hypoechoic plaque (*arrowhead*).

Diagnosis: Low-echogenicity plaque. Fibrofatty plaque is the least echogenic type of plaque and contains a large amount of lipid material. It may be so faintly echogenic that it is difficult to identify sonographically. The echogenicity of fibrofatty plaque is less than or equal to that of the sternocleidomastoid muscle. Problems in detecting hypoechoic plaque can be lessened with color flow imaging, because a flow void and possibly any flow disturbance are made visible, even if the plaque is not seen. The transverse view is of considerable importance for assessment of the thickness of the plaque and for visual measurement of luminal narrowing (6).

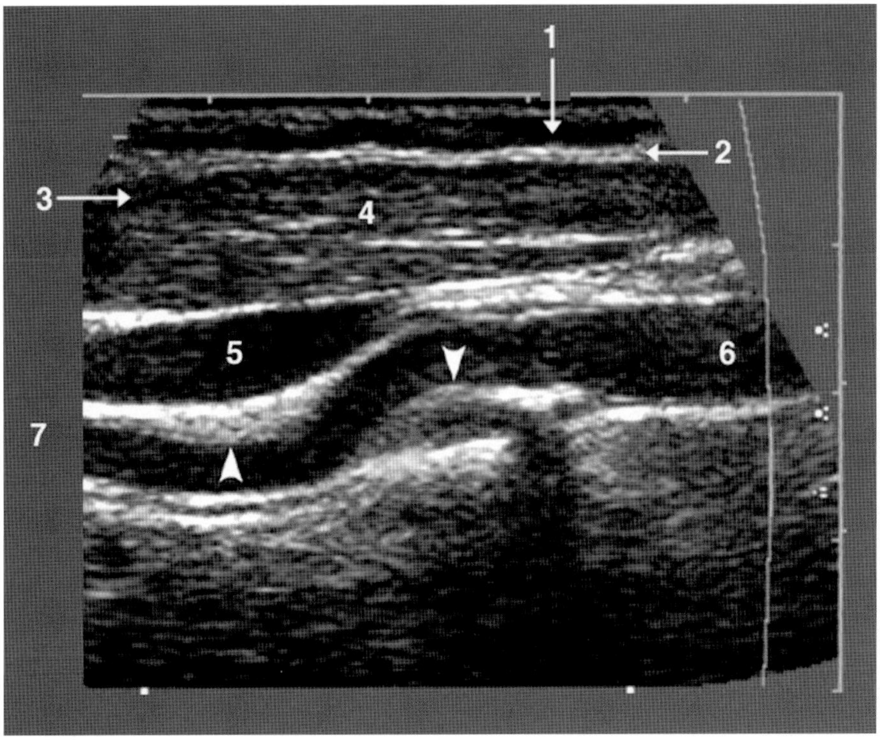

FIGURE 5.10. Right common and internal carotid arteries. Lateral view. Longitudinal. Gray scale. *1*, Skin and superficial cervical fascia; *2*, platysma; *3*, deep cervical fascia; *4*, sternocleidomastoid muscle; *5*, right internal jugular vein; *6*, right common carotid artery; *7*, right internal carotid artery; tandem plaques in the right carotid system (*arrowheads*).

Diagnosis: Tandem plaques in the carotid systems. Flow in a curved path in the circulatory system is so common that special emphasis on this type of flow is appropriate. For any case of curved flow, the pressure increases with radius and the velocity increases as the radius decreases. Secondary flow occurs in the flow around a bend in blood vessels. This secondary flow, which consists of two spirals, is superimposed upon the primary flow. The diminished lateral pressure on the convex surface of bends stimulates the endothelium to proliferate with a progressively thickened intima that provides the initial stimulus for the development of atherosclerosis (7).

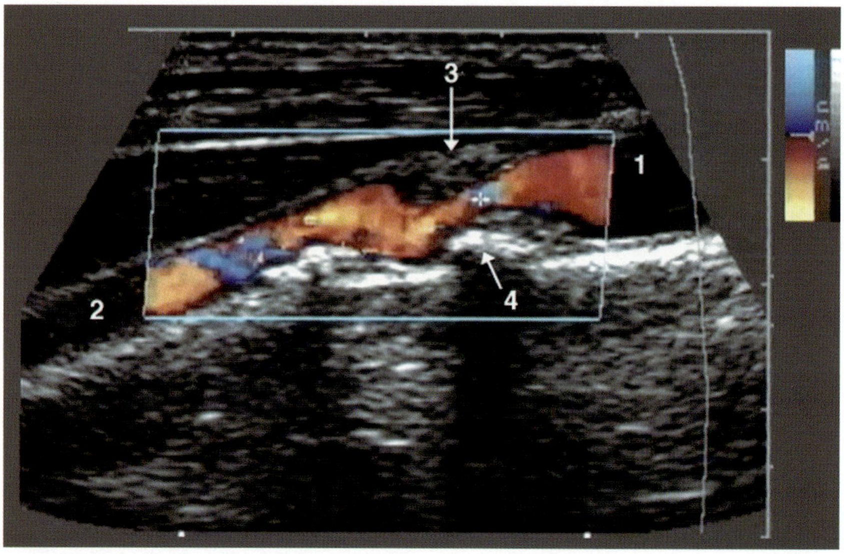

A

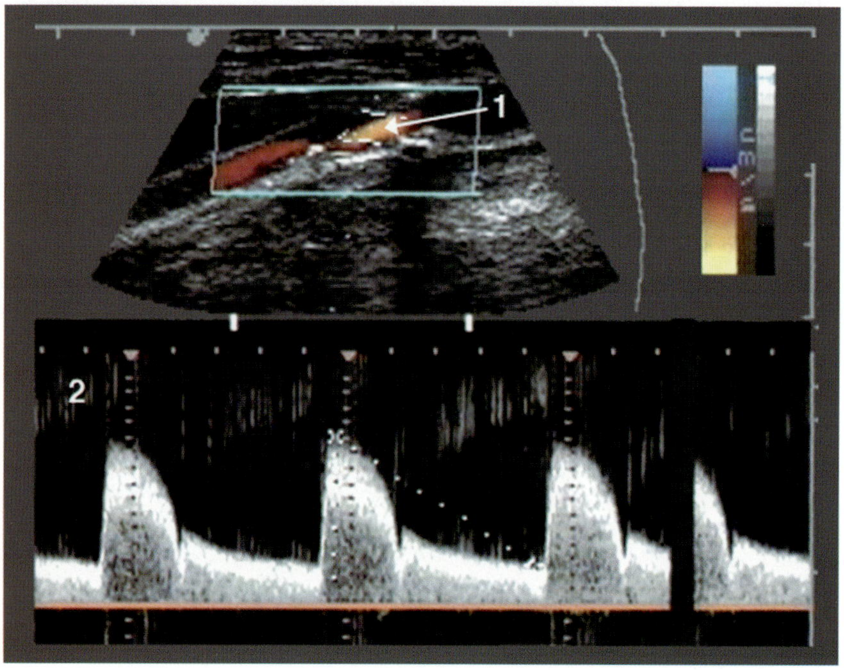

B

FIGURE 5.11. A: Right bifurcation of the common carotid artery and right internal carotid artery. Lateral view. Longitudinal. Color. *1*, Right common carotid artery; *2*, right internal carotid artery; *3*, soft plaque at the near wall of the bifurcation of the right common carotid artery; *4*, calcified plaque in the far wall of the bifurcation of the right common carotid artery with acoustic shadowing behind. **B:** Right bifurcation of the common carotid artery and right internal carotid artery. Lateral view. Longitudinal. Color. *1*, Sample placed at the jet of the stenosis; *2*, Doppler spectrum of the jet.

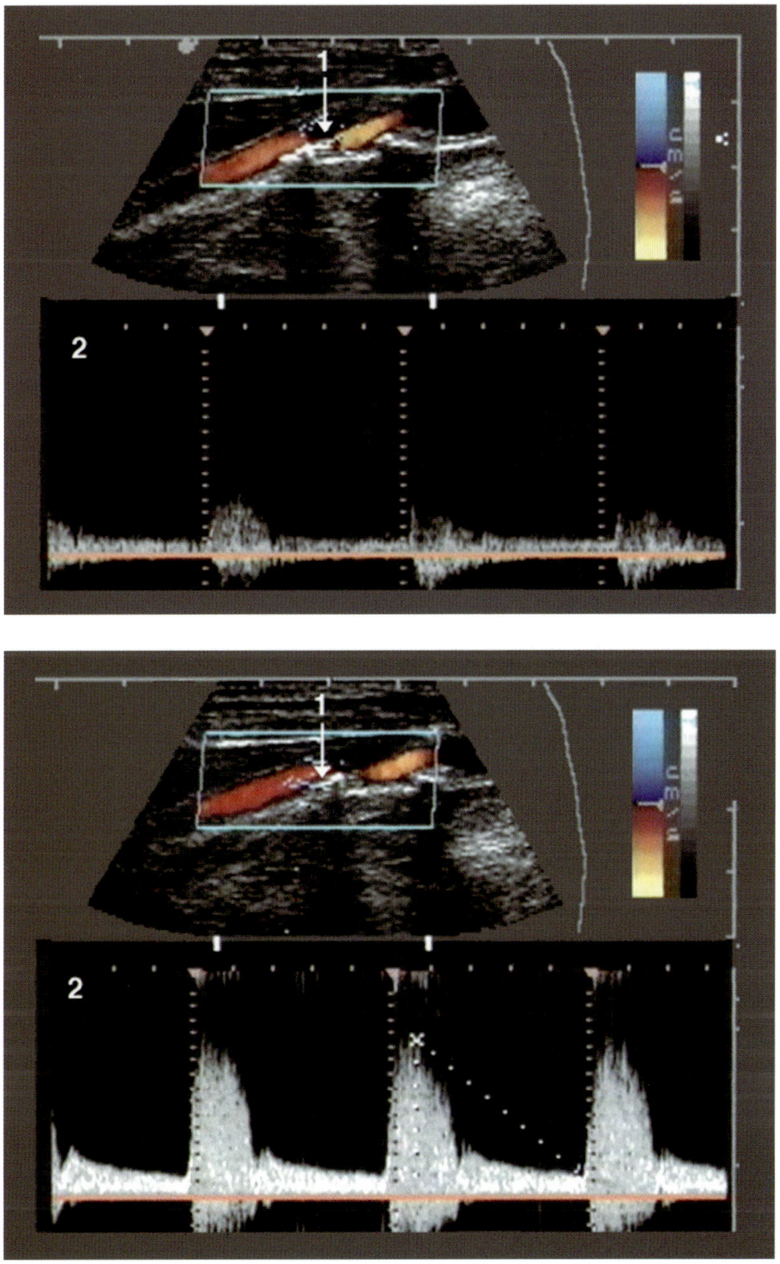

C

D

FIGURE 5.11. ***(continued)*** **C:** Right bifurcation of the common carotid artery and right internal carotid artery. Lateral view. Longitudinal. Color. *1*, Sample placed at the poststenotic turbulence; *2*, Doppler spectrum of the poststenotic turbulence. **D:** Right bifurcation of the common carotid artery and right internal carotid artery. Lateral view. Longitudinal. Color. *1*, Sample placed at the second stenotic jet; *2*, Doppler spectrum of the second stenotic jet.

Diagnosis: Tandem stenotic lesion of the right bifurcation and internal carotid artery. Changes in the direction of the bloodstream in the stenotic tandem lesions of the carotid arteries can be imaged by color mapping. The clinical uses of color flow imaging in these cases are that (a) it depicts flow dynamics over long segments of the carotid systems, (b) the sample can be placed over the stenotic jet, and (c) Doppler waveform analysis with appropriate Doppler angle correction can be done rapidly. Color flow imaging of the right carotid system with stenotic tandem lesion is shown in all views of the figure. Without the color map, the artery would be difficult to trace. The zones of increased velocity were rapidly localized and two clear hemodynamically stenotic jets were found. This is an example of one of the clinically relevant indications of color flow imaging of the carotid arteries (8).

PEARLS AND PITFALLS

Pearls

- B-mode examination allows the evaluation of plaque and its classification based on the echogenicity, structure, and surface characteristics.
- Calcification can be present in either form of plaque, homogenous or heterogenous, and does not enter into the scheme of classification.
- The transverse view is important to assess the thickness of the plaque and for visual measurement of luminal narrowing.
- Advantages of color-coded Doppler imaging include detection of hypoechoic plaque and better delineation of surface features of plaque.

Pitfalls

- Without color-coded Doppler sonography, a sonolucent area of intraplaque hemorrhage can be misdiagnosed as ulcerate plaque.
- Low-echodensity plaques or thrombus formation might go undetected on conventional B-mode imaging; however, color Doppler sonography gives an excellent delineation of such vessel wall irregularities.
- A single, longitudinal examination can easily miss atherosclerotic changes lateral to the plane section. Multiple scans are necessary.
- A heterogeneous lesion contains one or more well-defined hypoechoic areas that may represent intraplaque hemorrhage or other pathology. Acoustic shadowing can also cause this finding.

QUESTIONS

1. The classification of the plaque is based on the echo pattern assessed by two criteria: ________ and ________ .
   a. echogenicity, homogeneity
   b. echogenicity, calcifications
   c. homogeneity, calcifications
   d. brightness, calcifications
   e. echogenicity, brightness

2. The degree of uniformity of the echo pattern within the plaque compared with the soft tissues surrounding the vessel wall is called brightness.
   True or false?

3. Which of the following aspects do not enter into the scheme of classification of the carotid plaque with B-mode evaluation?
   a. Echogeneity
   b. Surface
   c. Calcifications
   d. Homogeneity
   e. Brightness

4. The local biologic change that evokes the development of atherosclerosis in the inner wall of an artery curvature is because, at that level, ________
   a. the flow velocity increases.
   b. the static pressure decreases.
   c. the flow velocity decreases.
   d. a and b
   e. b and c

5. As the radius decreases, the velocity ________ and the static pressure ________ in a curved flow.
   a. increases, increases
   b. decreases, decreases
   c. increases, decreases
   d. decreases, increases
   e. None of the above

6. The ability to identify ulcerations in arterial walls with ultrasound is well known, with a sensitivity of 90% and specificity of 100%.
   True or false?

7. The acoustic shadowing behind the brightly echogenic areas (Fig. 5.12) means that the plaque is calcified, changing the scheme of classification proposed by the European Carotid Plaque Study Group.
   True or false?

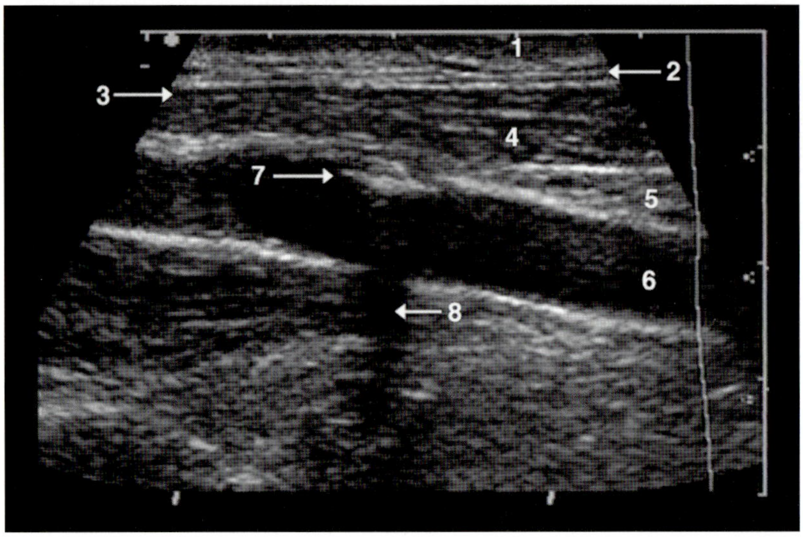

FIGURE 5.12. Bifurcation of the left common carotid artery. Lateral view. Gray scale. *1*, Skin and superficial cervical fascia; *2*, platysma; *3*, deep cervical fascia; *4*, sternocleidomastoid muscle; *5*, internal jugular vein; *6*, left common carotid artery; *7*, heterogeneous calcified plaque at the bifurcation of the left common carotid artery; *8*, acoustic shadowing resulting from calcific plaque.

8. A small calcified plaque formation is on the near wall of the common carotid artery (Fig. 5.13) with distal shadowing. As a result, no Doppler signal and no useful color flow information can be obtained.

True or false?

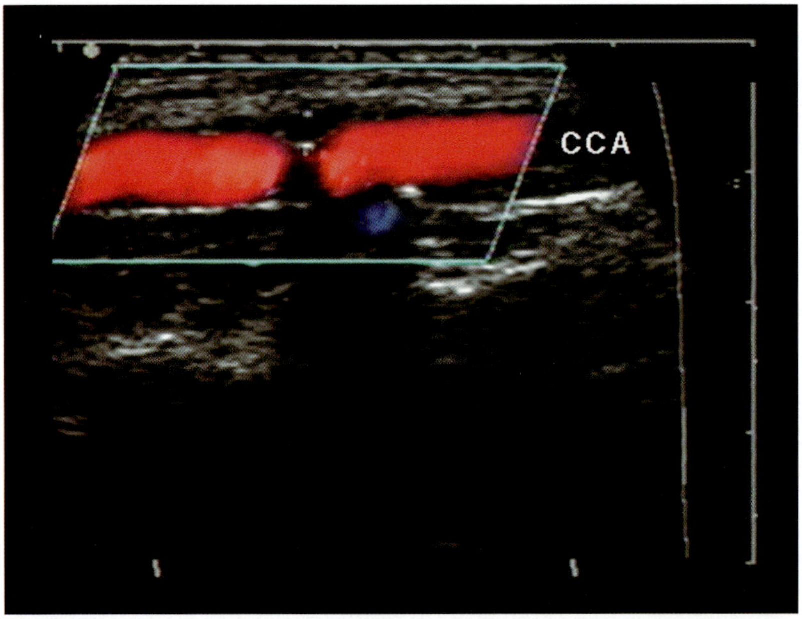

FIGURE 5.13. Right common carotid artery (CCA). Lateral view. Longitudinal. Color.

Answers: **1.** a; **2.** False; **3.** c; **4.** d; **5.** c; **6.** False; **7.** False; **8.** True.

REFERENCES

1. European Carotid Plaque Study Group. Carotid artery plaque composition. Relationship to clinical presentation and ultrasound B-mode imaging. *Eur J Vasc Endovasc Surg* 1995;10:23–30.
2. Texon M. *Hemodynamic basis of atherosclerosis.* Washington, DC: Hemisphere, 1980.
3. Bluth E, McVay L, Merrit C, et al. The identification of ulcerative plaque with high resolutions duplex carotid scanning. *J Ultrasound Med* 1988;1:73–76.
4. Bluth EI, Kay D, Merritt CRB, et al. Sonographic characterization of carotid plaque: detection of hemorrhage. *Am J Neuroradiol* 1986;7:311–314.
5. Tratting S, Hübsch P. Color-coded Doppler sonography of the carotid arteries. In: Frühwald F, Blackwell DE, eds. *Atlas of color-coded Doppler sonography: vascular and soft tissue structures of the upper extremity. Thoracic outlet and neck.* Vienna: Springer-Verlag, 1992.
6. Zwiebel WJ. Color-duplex features of normal and abnormal carotid arteries. In: Zwiebel WJ, ed. *Introduction to vascular ultrasonography,* 3rd ed. Philadelphia: WB Saunders, 1992.
7. Texon M. Hemodynamic basis of atherosclerosis. Washington, DC: McGraw-Hill, 1980.
8. Polak JF, Dobkin GR, O'Leary DH, et al. Internal carotid artery stenosis: accuracy and reproducibility of color Doppler assisted duplex imaging. *Radiology* 1989;173: 793–798.

CHAPTER 6

ANATOMIC VARIANTS AND CONGENITAL ABNORMALITIES OF THE EXTRACRANIAL CAROTID SYSTEM

In textbooks on anatomy, only the "normal" arterial blood supply is usually described. This so-called normality is sometimes found in less than 30% of cases for some arteries and in more than 95% for others.

The "abnormal" vascular patterns of the extracranial carotid system are being reported in increasing numbers. There has been a surge of clinical interest in the topographic anatomy of the arterial blood supply, the origin of arteries, and the area supplied by individual vessels. With angiography or Doppler ultrasonography, one can visualize *in vivo* many variations that were identified previously only in dissected anatomic preparations.

They can be classified into two groups: (a) anomalies or variations and (b) malformations. The anomalies or variations generally have no effect on the function of the organ under normal circumstances and are asymptomatic. The malformations, in contrast, have a negative influence on the function of the organ under normal circumstances.

Classification of arterial variations is usually based on normal embryologic development.

The following cases demonstrate the most common arterial anomalies found in duplex scanning studies and their clinical implications.

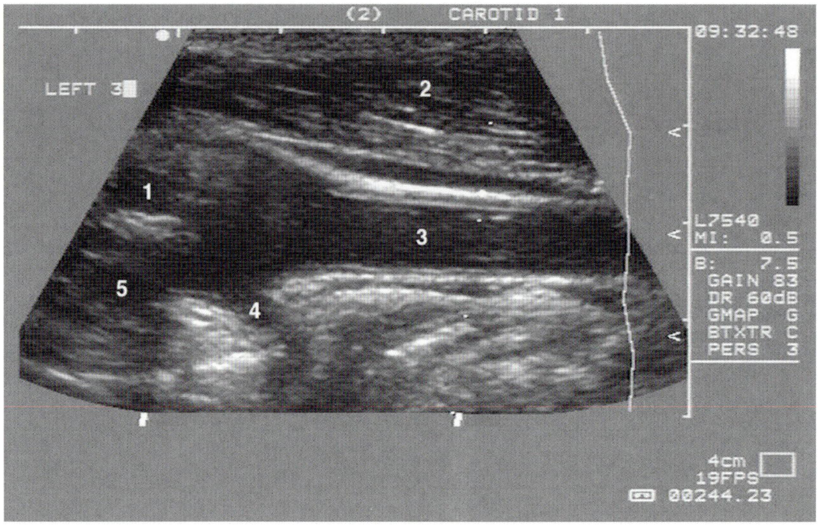

FIGURE 6.1. Bifurcation of the left common carotid artery. Posterolateral view. Longitudinal. Gray scale. *1*, Left internal carotid artery; *2*, sternocleidomastoid muscle; *3*, left common carotid artery; *4*, left superior thyroid artery (originates from bifurcation); *5*, left external carotid artery.

Diagnosis: The superior thyroid artery originates from the bifurcation of the common carotid artery. The external carotid artery originates from the common carotid artery at the midcervical level and is the smaller of its two terminal branches. The superior thyroid artery is the first anterior branch of the external carotid artery and supplies the larynx and superior pole of the thyroid gland. It courses inferiorly, lying parallel and anterior to the common carotid artery. The superior thyroid artery originates from the bifurcation of the common carotid in 20% of cases, and it is more frequent on the left than on the right side (1).

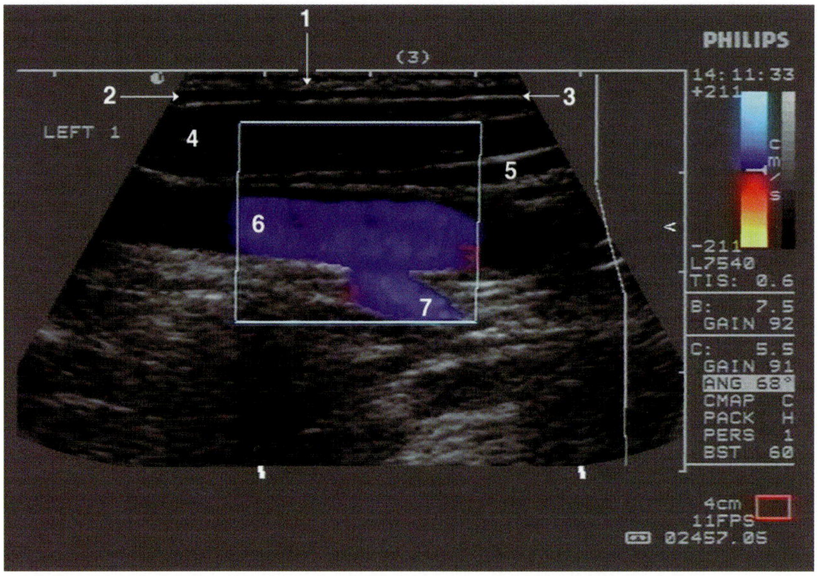

FIGURE 6.2. Left common carotid artery. Anteroposterior view. Longitudinal. Color. *1*, Skin and superficial cervical fascia; *2*, platysma; *3*, deep cervical fascia; *4*, sternocleidomastoid muscle; *5*, left internal jugular vein; *6*, left common carotid artery; *7*, overloaded color in a branch of thyrocervical trunk.

Diagnosis: The superior thyroid artery originates from the common carotid artery. In 10% of the cases, the superior thyroid artery originates from the common carotid artery. This is true in females more often than in males, and it is on the left side more often than on the right. In this figure, if it should be a branch of the common carotid artery, the color flow imaging should show a red color in it (1).

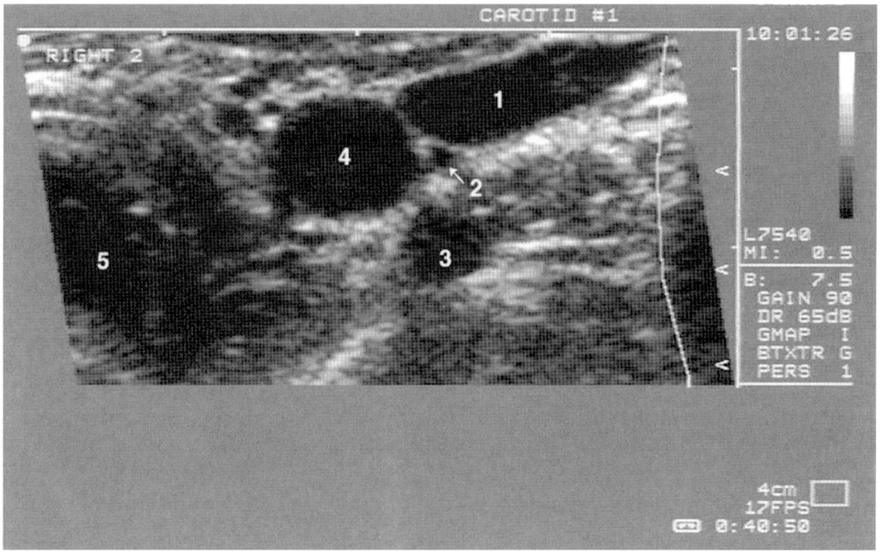

FIGURE 6.3. Bifurcation of the right common carotid artery. Transverse view. Gray scale. *1*, Right internal jugular vein; *2*, vagus nerve; *3*, right external carotid artery; *4*, right internal carotid artery; *5*, trachea.

Diagnosis: Carotid bifurcation. Prendes anomaly. An anatomic variant for the position of the external carotid artery (ECA) is present at the carotid bifurcation.The ECA is lateral to and posterior to the internal carotid artery. This anomaly can be noted in 5% of the patients studied by Doppler ultrasound (2).

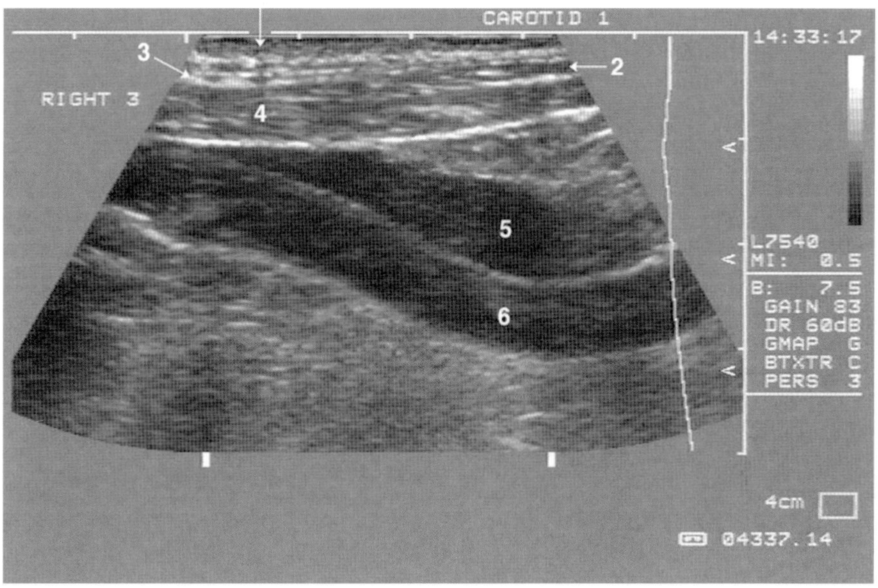

FIGURE 6.4. Right common carotid artery. Posterolateral view. Longitudinal. Gray scale. *1*, Skin and superficial cervical fascia; *2*, platysma; *3*, deep cervical fascia; *4*, sternocleidomastoid muscle; *5*, right internal jugular vein; *6*, right common carotid artery.

Diagnosis: Tortuosity of the common carotid artery. There is a discrepancy in the terminology of this anomaly and some authors have suggested the following definitions: tortuosity—any S-shaped or C-shaped elongation or undulation in the course of the artery; coiling—elongation of the artery resulting in an exaggerated S-shaped curve or in a circular configuration; kinking—angulation of one or more segments of the artery associated with stenosis in the affected segment. These anomalies may be present in childhood, but they may increase with age. Kinking is thought to be an acquired condition resulting from arteriosclerosis (3).

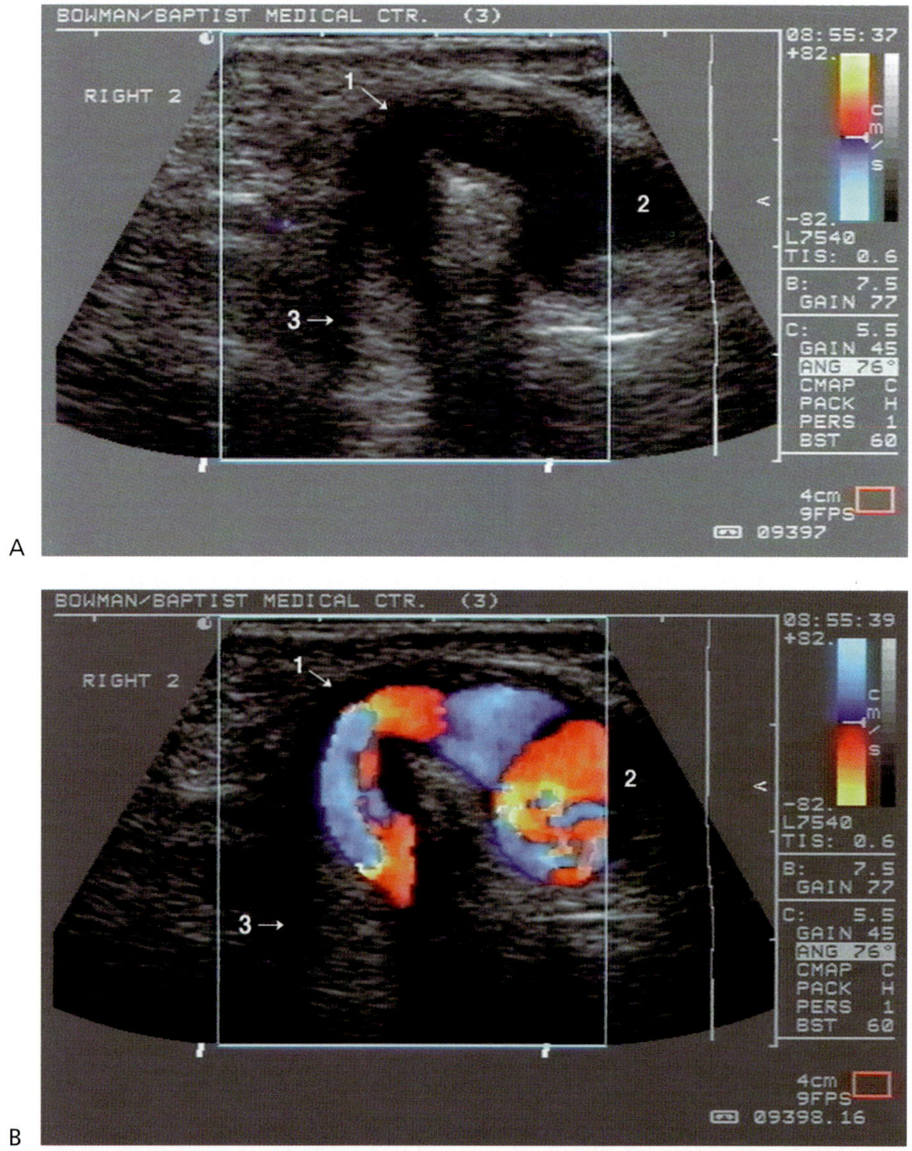

FIGURE 6.5. Right common carotid artery. Lateral view. Longitudinal. Gray scale **(A)** and color **(B)**. *1*, Semicircular shape of right carotid artery; *2*, right common carotid artery buckle from coiling; *3*, refraction (edge) shadowing.

Diagnosis: Coiling of the common carotid artery. Angulation of the common carotid artery usually occurs on the right side. Proximally, the right common carotid is relatively fixed at its origin from the innominate artery and is a continuation of the ascending aorta. It is directly subjected to the systolic impulse that may accentuate the mechanical consequence of elevation of the aortic arch. Usually a buckle of the common carotid artery requires no specific therapy, and some authors agree that surgery is only indicated in highly selective cases to correct a kink (4).

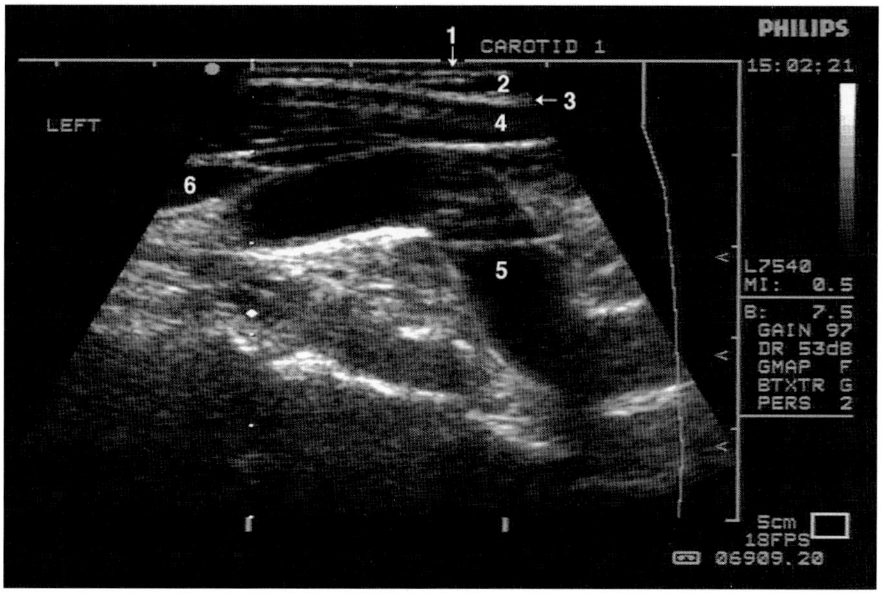

FIGURE 6.6. Left common carotid artery. Lateral view. Longitudinal. Gray scale. *1*, Skin and superficial cervical fascia; *2*, platysma; *3*, deep cervical fascia; *4*, sternocleidomastoid muscle; *5*, left common carotid artery, kinking; *6*, left internal jugular vein.

Diagnosis: Kinking of the common carotid artery. The significance of elongation of the carotid artery is controversial. In general, the term *carotid artery tortuosity* has been applied to angulations of markedly different severity, and angulation of common carotid or cervical internal carotid arteries has not been differentiated. As a result, indications for surgical treatment are not uniform, and some patients may have been needlessly exposed to the risks of a major operation. Angulation of the common carotid artery usually occurs on the right side. The right common carotid artery is an approximate continuation of the ascending aorta and is directly subject to the systolic impulse. Hypertension and atherosclerotic vascular disease contribute to elevation of the aortic arch and the subsequent formation of a kink in the common carotid artery (5).

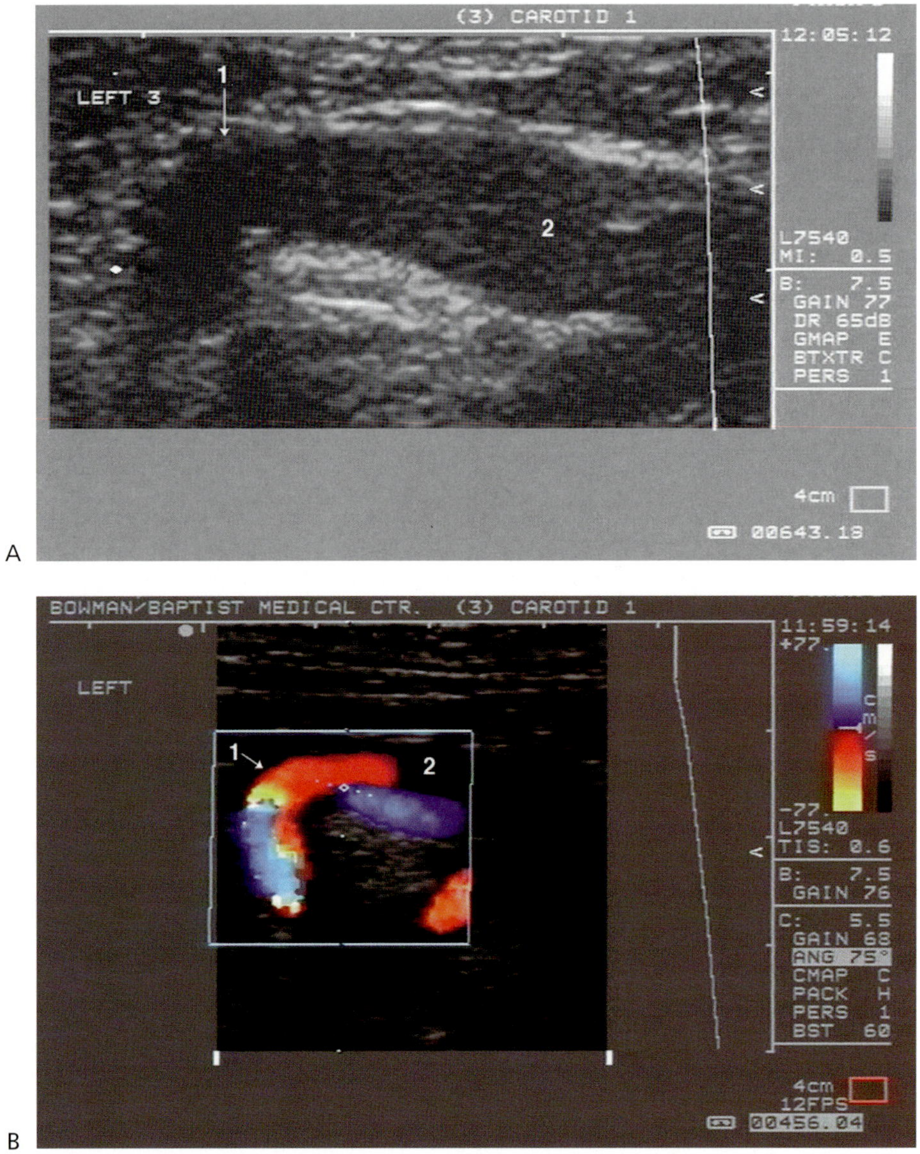

FIGURE 6.7. Left internal carotid artery. Posterolateral view. Longitudinal. Gray scale **(A)** and color **(B)**. *1*, Angulation grade I of Metz's classification; *2*, left internal carotid artery.

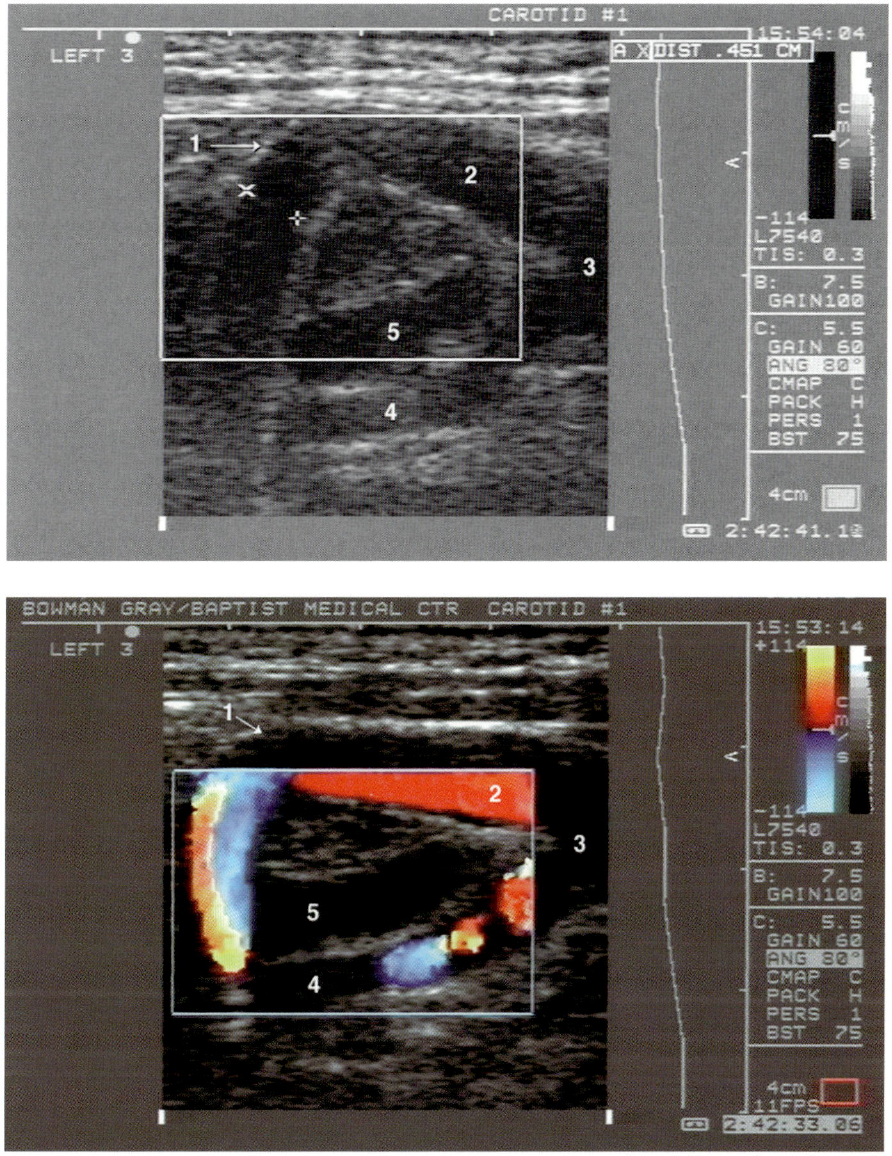

A

B

FIGURE 6.8. Bifurcation of the left common carotid artery. Posterolateral view. Longitudinal. Gray scale **(A)** and color **(B)**. *1*, Angulation grade I of Metz's classification; *2*, left internal carotid artery; *3*, bifurcation of the left common carotid artery; *4*, left external carotid artery; *5*, left internal jugular vein.

Diagnosis: Tortuosity of the internal carotid artery. (Metz grade I). Unlike the common carotid artery, the internal carotid artery on each side has a fairly similar course and occasionally gentle curves are noted in it. A great deal of confusion has surrounded the broadly descriptive terms used to classify any irregularity in the path of the vessel. Metz and coworkers were the first group to analyze these lesions in a quantitative manner. According to Metz's classification of angulations of the internal carotid artery, in a grade I abnormality, the acute angle between the two segments is 90 to 60 degrees. The angle of a grade II angulation lies between 60 and 30 degrees. The angle of a grade III irregularity is less than 30 degrees. These authors included complete loops of the internal carotid artery in the original grade III. A kink of the internal carotid would correspond to its class III abnormality, and such lesions have potential clinical importance (6).

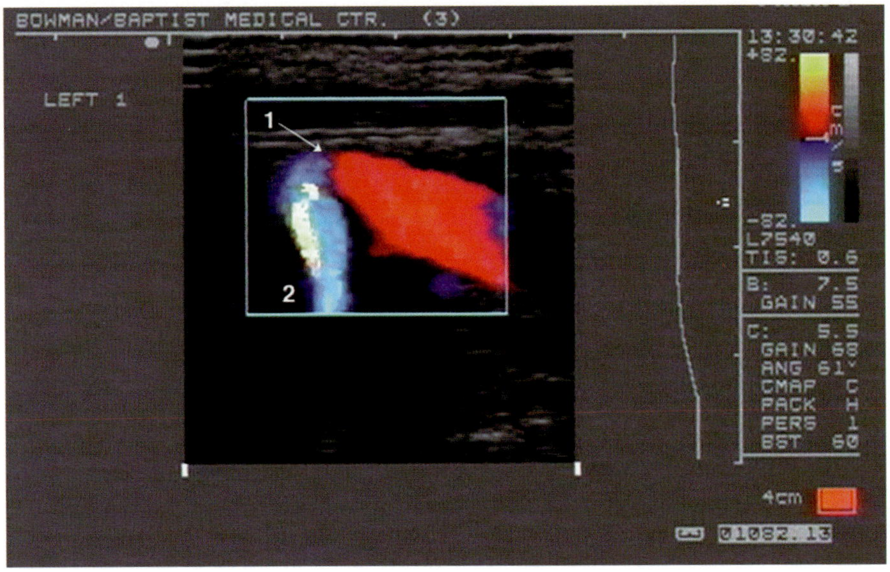

FIGURE 6.9. Left internal carotid artery. Anteroposterior view. Longitudinal. Color. *1*, Angulation grade II of Metz's classification; *2*, left internal carotid artery.

Diagnosis: Tortuosity of the internal carotid artery (Metz grade II). Several theories regarding the origin of tortuosity of the internal carotid artery have been refuted, and a developmental etiology based on the concept of persistent fetal angulation has been widely accepted and supported by the occurrence of tortuosity of common carotid in young patients, bilaterally and without atherosclerotic vascular disease (7).

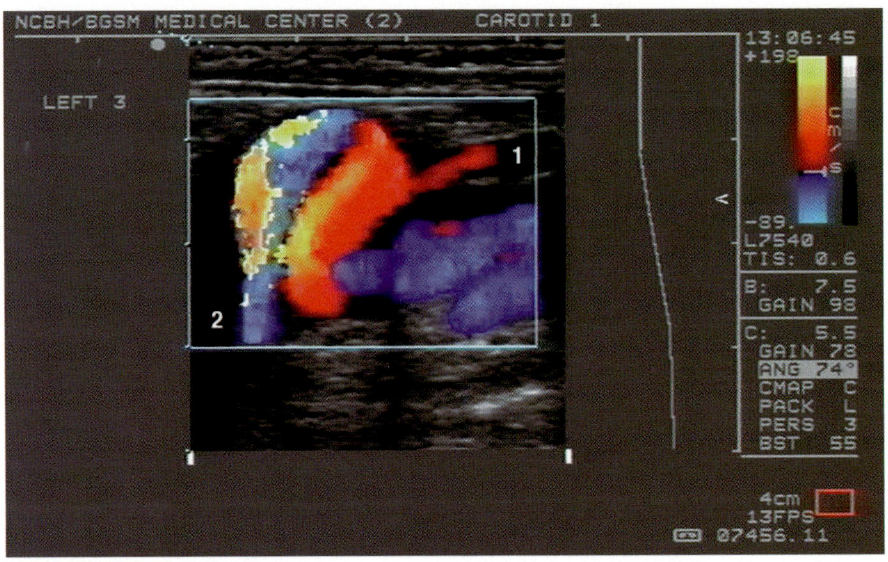

FIGURE 6.10. Left internal carotid artery. Posterolateral view. Longitudinal. Color. *1*, Left internal jugular vein; *2*, left internal carotid artery.

Diagnosis: Kinking of the internal carotid artery (Metz grade III). A grade III abnormality of Metz's classification corresponds to a kink of the internal carotid artery (ICA). Whereas tortuosity of the ICA is essentially a congenital problem, kinking may represent an acquired condition. Atherosclerotic vascular disease and senile degenerative changes with elastic tissue destruction may contribute to the kink. Kinks of the ICA may cause ischemic symptoms. Only when other etiologic possibilities have been excluded, should it be accepted as the cause of cerebrovascular insufficiency with surgery recommended (8).

PEARLS AND PITFALLS

Pearls

- Tortuosity, coiling, and kinking of the common carotid artery may be present in childhood. Kinking is regarded to be a more acquired condition resulting from arteriosclerosis.
- Angulation of the common carotid artery usually occurs on the right side where it is directly subjected to the systolic impulse that accentuates the mechanical elevation of the aortic arch.
- A kink of the internal carotid artery or a class III abnormality of Metz's classification has potential clinical importance.

Pitfalls

- In a carotid Doppler scan, the vessel imaged anteriorly in the carotid bifurcation can be misidentified as the external carotid artery (Prendes anomaly).
- It is necessary to exclude other etiologic possibilities to avoid a misdiagnosis of cerebrovascular insufficiency caused by a kink of the internal carotid artery.
- In case of tortuosity of the internal carotid artery, a close probe-to-vessel angle insonation in Doppler sonography would cause misinterpretation as stenotic flow because of the false increase in blood flow velocity recording.
- Imaging of the superior thyroid artery from the bifurcation with conventional gray scale could be a source of error to identify the external carotid artery based on its branches.

QUESTIONS

1. The superior thyroid artery
   a. is the first branch of the internal carotid artery.
   b. can arise from the bifurcation in about 70% of the cases.
   c. supplies the larynx and superior pole of the thyroid gland.
   d. All of the above
   e. None of the above

2. The superior thyroid artery originates from the bifurcation of the common carotid artery in 20% of the cases, and it is more frequent on the left than the right side.
   True or false?

3. The superior thyroid artery originates from the common carotid artery
   a. more frequently than from the bifurcation.
   b. more often in males.
   c. more often on the right side.
   d. All of the above
   e. None of the above

4. The Prendes anomaly
   a. is an anatomic variant for the position of the internal carotid artery.
   b. is always bilateral.
   c. supplies the face by the internal carotid artery.
   d. All of the above
   e. None of the above

5. In the anatomic variant known as the Prendes anomaly, the external carotid artery is ________ and ________ to the internal carotid artery.
   a. lateral, posterior
   b. lateral, anterior
   c. medial, anterior
   d. medial, posterior
   e. None of the above

6. Any S-shaped or C-shaped elongation or undulation in the course of the artery is called ________ .
   a. elongation
   b. tortuosity
   c. angulation
   d. coiling
   e. kinking

7. Any elongation of the artery resulting in an exaggerated S-shaped curve or in circular configuration is called ________ .
   a. elongation
   b. tortuosity
   c. angulation
   d. coiling
   e. kinking

8. Any angulation of one or more segments of the artery with stenosis in the affected segment is called ________ .
    a. elongation
    b. tortuosity
    c. angulation
    d. coiling
    e. kinking

9. In relation to tortuosity, coiling, and kinking,
    a. they may be present in childhood.
    b. they may be increased with age.
    c. the latter is thought to be an acquired condition caused by arteriosclerosis.
    d. All of the above
    e. None of the above

10. The angulations of the common carotid artery
    a. usually occur on the left side.
    b. always require surgical therapy.
    c. are buckles of the common carotid artery and usually require no specific therapy.
    d. All of the above
    e. None of the above

11. Angulations of the common carotid artery usually occur on the right side because the right common carotid artery is an approximate continuation of the ascending aorta, and it is subjected to the mechanical consequence of the elevation of the aortic arch with the systolic pulse.

    True or false?

12. In relation to angulations of the common carotid artery,
    a. indications for surgical therapy are not uniform.
    b. hypertension is a risk factor.
    c. atherosclerotic vascular disease is a risk factor.
    d. All of the above
    e. None of the above

13. According to Metz's classification of angulations of the internal carotid artery, match the different grades of angulations with the angles measured between the two segments of the artery.

1. Grade I abnormality	a. The angle is less than 30 degrees.
2. Grade II abnormality	b. Angle lies between 30 and 60 degrees.
3. Grade III abnormality	c. Angle lies between 60 and 90 degrees.

14. A developmental etiology of fetal origin of the angulation of the internal carotid artery is supported by the occurrence of tortuosity in young patients, bilaterally and without atherosclerotic vascular disease.

    True or false?

15. Kinking of the internal carotid artery may represent
    a. a congenital condition.
    b. an inherited condition.
    c. an acquired condition.
    d. All of the above
    e. None of the above

16. The kinks of the internal carotid artery
    a. correspond to a class II abnormality of Metz's classification.
    b. may be a cause of ischemic symptoms.
    c. always lead to surgical therapy.
    d. All of the above
    e. None of the above

Answers: **1.** c; **2.** True; **3.** e; **4.** e; **5.** a; **6.** b; **7.** d; **8.** e; **9.** d; **10.** c; **11.** True; **12.** d; **13.** 1c, 2b, 3a; **14.** True; **15.** c; **16.** b.

REFERENCES

1. Lippert H, Pabst R. Arterial variations in man. Classification and frequency. J F Bergmann Verlag, Munchen 1985.
2. Prendes JL, McKinney WM, Buonanno FS, et al. Anatomic variations of the carotid bifurcation affecting Doppler scan interpretation. J Clin Ultrasound 1980;8:147–150.
3. Lie TA. Congenital malformations of the carotid and vertebral arterial systems, including the persistent anastomoses. In: Vinken PJ, Bruyn GW, eds. Vascular diseases of the nervous system. Handbook of Neurology. Amsterdam: North-Holland, 1972.
4. Kia-Nowry M. Common carotid kinking and cerebral insufficiency. Int Surg 1973;58: 646–647.
5. Leipzig TJ, Dohrmann GJ. The tortuous or kinked carotid artery: pathogenesis and clinical considerations. A historical review. Surg Neurol 1986;25:478–486.
6. Metz H, Murray-Leslie RM, Bannister RG, et al. Kinking of the internal carotid artery in relation to cerebrovascular disease. Lancet 1961;i:424–426.
7. Rundles WR, Kimble FD. The kinked carotid syndrome. Angiology 1969;20:177–194.
8. Stanton PE Jr, McChisky DA Jr, Lamis PA. Hemodynamic assessment and surgical correction of kinking of the internal carotid artery. Surgery 1978;84:793–802.

CHAPTER 7

INTERPRETATION OF TYPICAL ABNORMAL PULSES AND ALTERATION OF THE CARDIAC RHYTHM

The arterial pulse is the most fundamental sign of a clinician's and a basic part of a clinician's physical examination.

The arterial pulse is any periodic fluctuation that is caused by heart contraction and occurs at the same frequency. Whereas "the pulse" can refer to any pulsation, the flow pulsation in an artery is the longitudinal movement of blood that occurs with each beat of the heart.

An arterial pulsation is essentially a bounding wave of blood with varying vigor that diminishes with increasing distance from the heart. Of all the arterial pulses, the carotids are easily accessible and closest to the cardiac source and therefore most useful in evaluating heart activity.

Flow in an artery cannot be appreciated by inspection, however, pulsatile flow can be recorded when a Doppler ultrasonic probe is applied over the artery.

The characteristics of arterial pulses can indicate heart rate and rhythm, pulse contour (waveform), amplitude (strength), symmetry, and sometimes obstructions to blood flow.

The contour of the pulse wave has a smooth, rounded, or domed shape. Attention should be paid to the ascending portion, the peak, and the descending portion. Each wave crest should be compared with the next to detect cyclic differences.

The following cases define the most common types of pulse abnormalities.

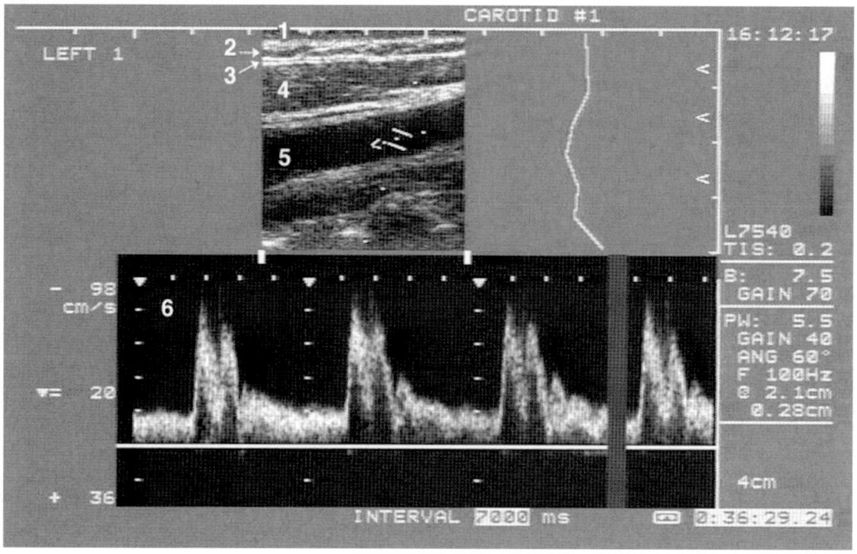

FIGURE 7.1. Right common carotid artery. Lateral view. Longitudinal. Gray scale and Doppler spectrum. *1*, Skin and superficial cervical fascia; *2*, platysma; *3*, deep cervical fascia; *4*, sternocleidomastoid muscle; *5*, right common carotid artery; *6*, Doppler spectrum shows bisferious pulse.

Diagnosis: Typical abnormal pulse. Bisferious pulse. Based on the glossary of cardiologic terms on the pulse published by the Committee on Standardized Terminology of the American College of Cardiology and the American Heart Association, the bisferious pulse is a pulse with two systolic peaks. Either the first or the second peak may be the highest, and differentiation based on this criterion may help to discern the etiology of the pulse. It is best palpated at the carotid artery and can occur in hypertrophic cardiomyopathy and mixed aortic stenosis and incompetence. In the bisferious pulse of hypertrophic cardiomyopathy, the initial pressure upstroke is brisk and the initial systolic wave is wider and of greater amplitude. This initial wave is followed by a relatively wide trough before the second systolic wave, which is usually of similar or lower amplitude than the first (1).

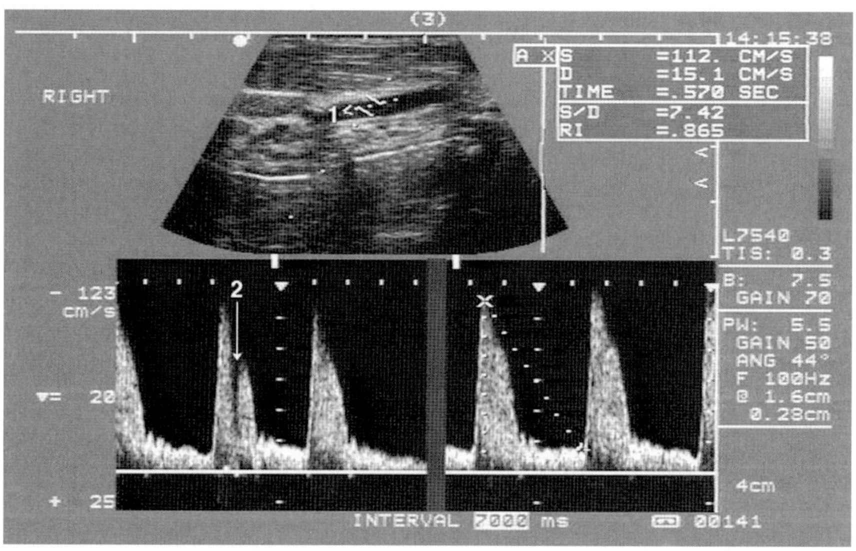

FIGURE 7.2. Right external carotid artery. Lateral view. Longitudinal. Gray scale. Doppler spectrum. *1*, Right external carotid artery; *2*, Doppler spectrum shows the midsystolic dipping in the second recorded beat. Brockenbrough phenomenon.

Diagnosis: Typical abnormal pulse. Bisferious pulse. In patients with hypertrophic obstructive cardiomyopathy (HOCM) without intraventricular gradient at rest, the midsystolic dipping occurred only in beats following extrasystoles. This finding is characteristic of HOCM and has been called the *Brockenbrough phenomenon*. An extrasystole increases the end diastolic volume and leads to enhanced contractility in the next regular beat (Frank-Starling mechanism). In patients with HOCM, an increase in contractility also increases the obstruction to ventricular outflow. Some transitory alteration in the intraventricular gradient resulting from a change in the heart rate could allow the characteristic change in the systolic component of the pulse in the patient shown (2).

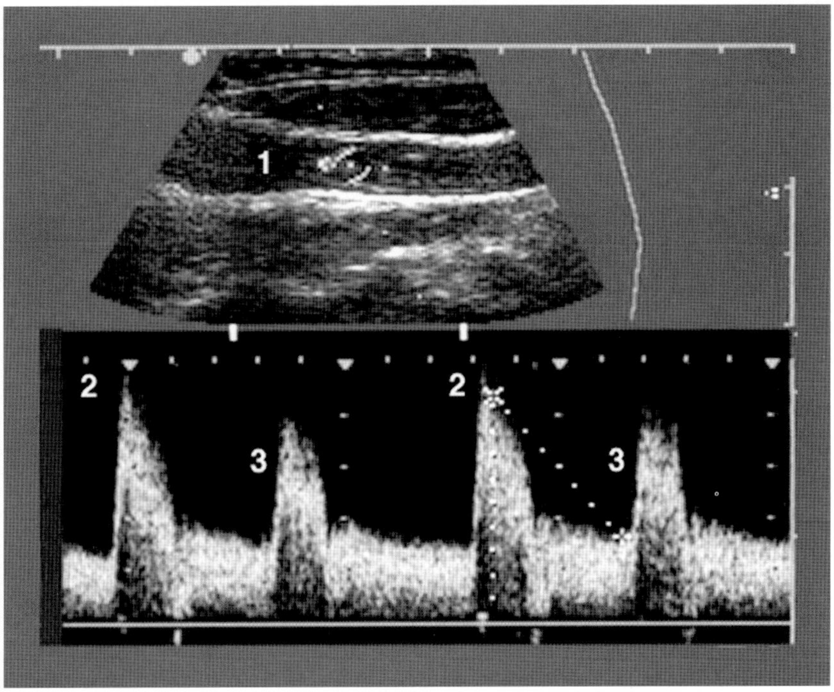

FIGURE 7.3. Left common carotid artery. Lateral view. Longitudinal. Gray scale. Doppler spectrum. *1*, Left common carotid artery; *2*, *3*, Doppler spectrum shows pulsus alternans.

Diagnosis: Pulsus alternans. Pulsus alternans is defined as a pulse pattern in which the beats occur at constant intervals, but with regular alternation of the peak of the pressure pulse or the rate of rise of the ascending limb. It differs from bisferious and dictoric pulses in that strong and weak pulses occur in consecutive beats with the heart contracting in a regular rhythm. Pulsus alternans usually indicates left ventricular failure (3).

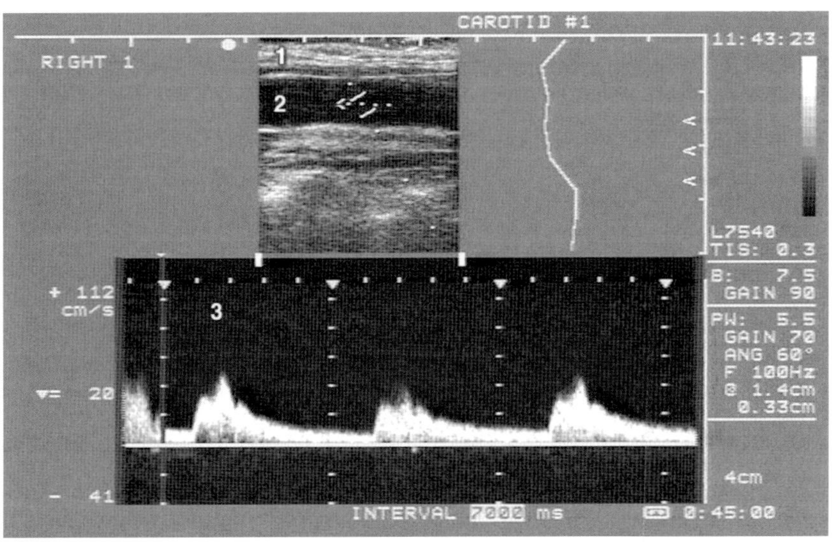

FIGURE 7.4. Right common carotid artery. Anteroposterior view. Longitudinal. Gray scale. Doppler spectrum. *1*, Sternocleidomastoid muscle; *2*, right common carotid artery; *3*, Doppler spectrum shows bisferious pulse.

Diagnosis: Mixed aortic stenosis and incompetence. The combined lesion of the aortic valve (stenosis and incompetence) usually produces one of the most distinctive pulses to be seen and felt in clinical practice. The pressure wave, in the ascending aorta, rises to an early systolic peak. Then, instead of rising slowly to a late systolic peak, as in aortic stenosis, it drops to a minimal value that corresponds with the peak of ejection from the left ventricle. Following this, the pressure rises to a late systolic peak. The first systolic peak is always lower than the second peak in late systole. This feature distinguishes the bisferious pulse of organic aortic valve disease from the bisferious pulse in hypertrophic cardiomyopathy (3).

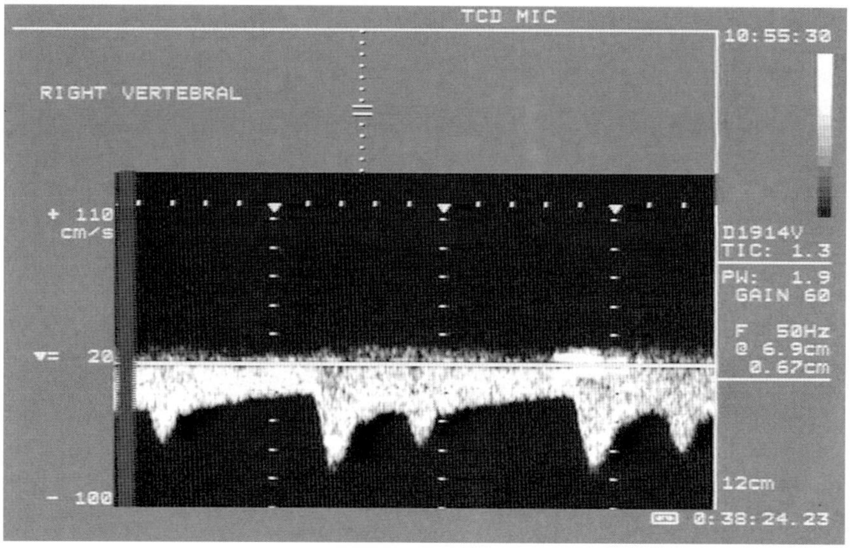

FIGURE 7.5. Transcranial Doppler sonography. Spectrum of the right vertebral artery via transforaminal approach.

Diagnosis: Typical abnormal pulse. Bigeminal pulse. In the pattern of bigeminal pulse, there is a regular coupling of two beats with the interval between a pair of beats greater than between the coupled beats themselves. The second weaker beat of each couple is usually produced by a premature ectopic beat coupled to a sinus beat with or without a compensatory pause. It may also be produced by others mechanism such as 3:2 Wenckebach atrioventricular block and nonconducted atrial premature systole following every second sinus beat (4).

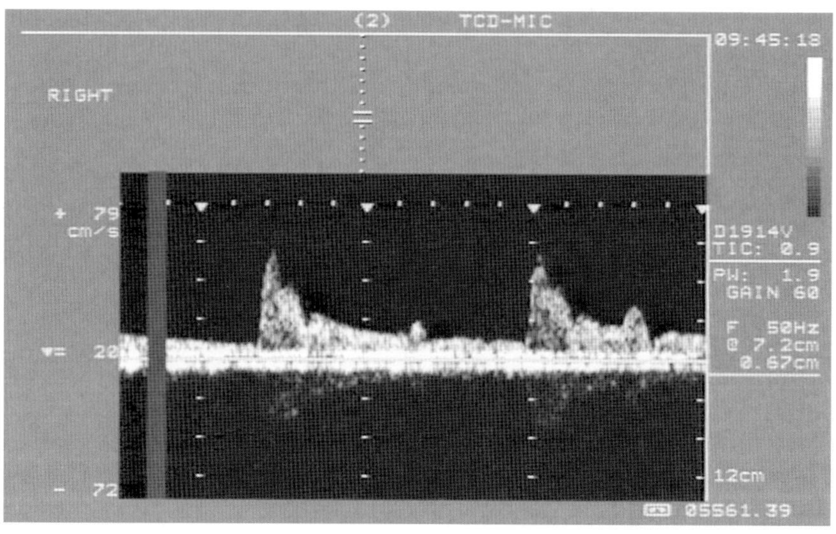

FIGURE 7.6. Transcranial Doppler sonography. Spectrum of the right middle cerebral artery.

Diagnosis: Arterial pulse in cardiovascular disease; atrial fibrillation. Having discussed abnormal pulse in particular conditions, it is appropriate to consider the types of pulses that one might expect to see in different cardiac arrhythmias. The mechanisms of these alterations can be explained on the basis of three principal factors: period of ejection from the heart, intensity of wave reflection, and timing of wave reflection. The nature of cardiac arrhythmias can often be diagnosed from the characteristics of the pulse. This is most apparent in atrial fibrillation in which sequential pulses are never the same (5).

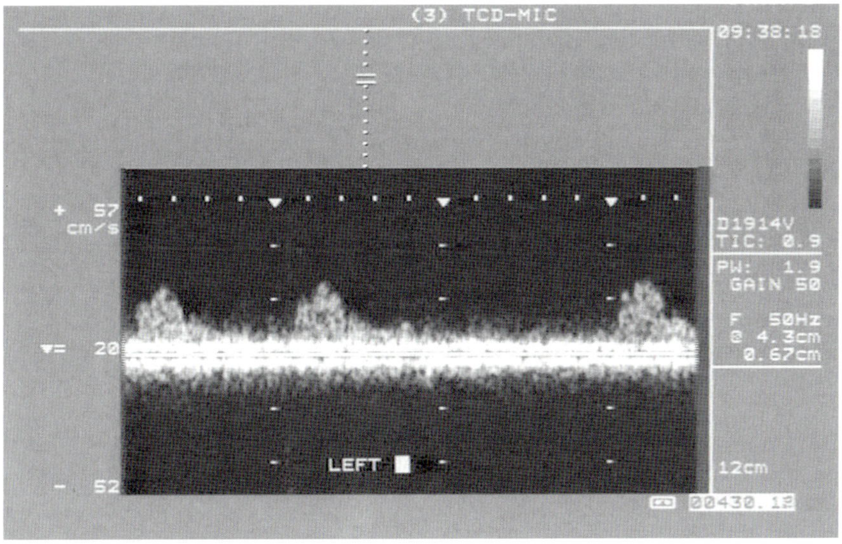

FIGURE 7.7. Transcranial Doppler sonography. Spectrum of the left ophthalmic artery showing the absence of the third beat.

Diagnosis: Surgical valvular implant. Sinus arrest. The sinus node can fail to stimulate the atria for one or more beats. This dysfunction may occur intermittently, with simply a missed beat at occasional intervals, or it may be more extreme. Abnormalities of the sinus node function are common in patients with atrial septal defect, after surgery, and with the use of calcium channel blockers (6).

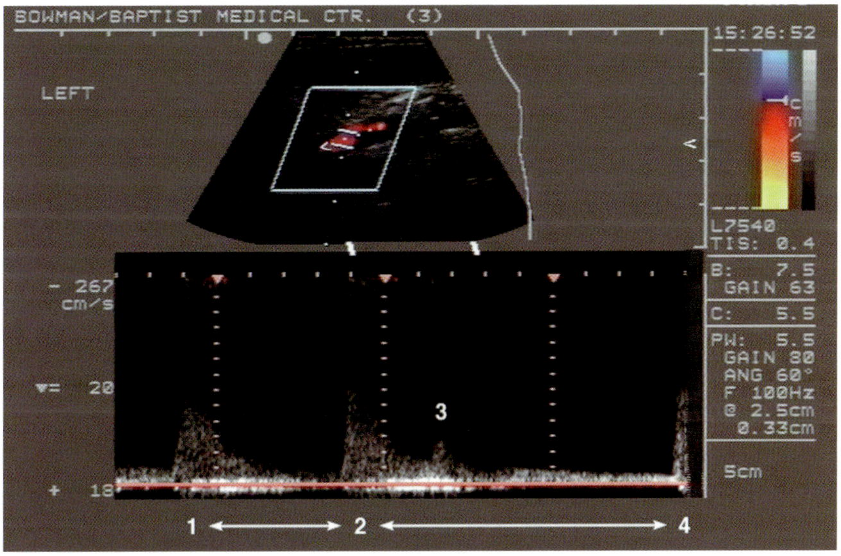

FIGURE 7.8. Left internal carotid artery. Lateral view. Longitudinal. Color. Doppler spectrum. The distance between the beats numbered *2* and *4* is double the distance between the beats numbered *1* and *2* (full compensatory pause). *3*, Ventricular premature beat.

Diagnosis: Ventricular premature beats (fully compensatory pause). Ectopic beats are often premature and may be atrial premature beats (APBs), atrioventricular premature beats (JPBs), or ventricular premature beats (VPBs). APBs and VPBs are usually followed by a pause before the next normal beat. A full compensatory pause indicates that the interval between the normal beat immediately before and immediately after the VPB is exactly twice the basal interval. This is the case in this figure. A full compensatory pause is more characteristic of VPBs (7).

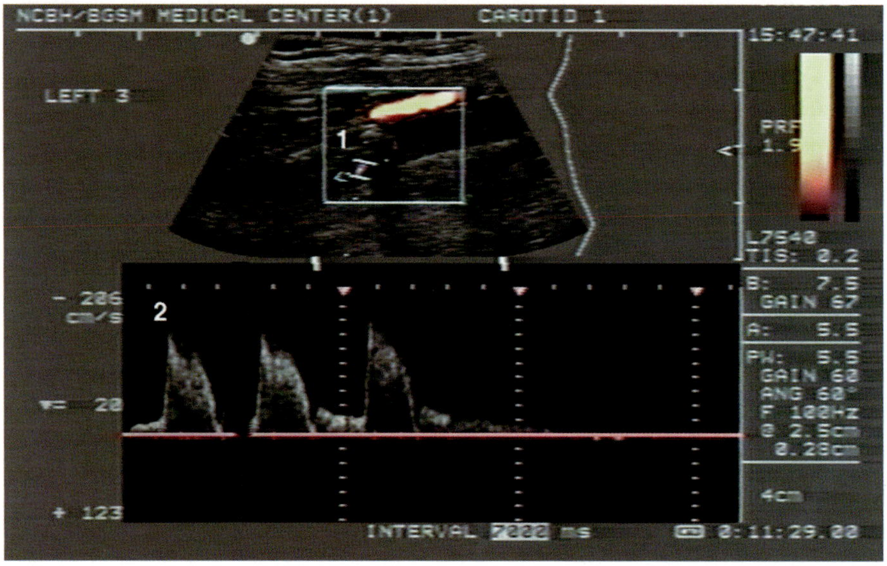

FIGURE 7.9. Left internal carotid artery. Anteroposterior view. Longitudinal. Gray scale. Doppler spectrum. Long pause asystole after carotid sinus stimulation by the transducer. *1*, Doppler sample was placed at the left external carotid artery; *2*, Doppler spectrum shows a long pause asystole after carotid sinus stimulation by the transducer.

Diagnosis: Carotid sinus hypersensitivity. Carotid sinus hypersensitivity (CSH) can cause stroke, cardiac asystole, and ventricular arrhythmias, but no predictors for CSH have been described. Duplex ultrasound is routinely used to study the carotid arteries and allows real-time wall motion assessment. The abnormal borderline response has been considered present if cardiac asystole lasted 2 seconds or more and if the heart rate decreased by 30% to 50%. Some authors have found a prevalence of 1.2% of hyperactive carotid sinus reflex in patients undergoing duplex sonography. Abnormal carotid artery wall motion, as longitudinal pulsation and loss of radial motion, have been described in these patients (8).

A

B

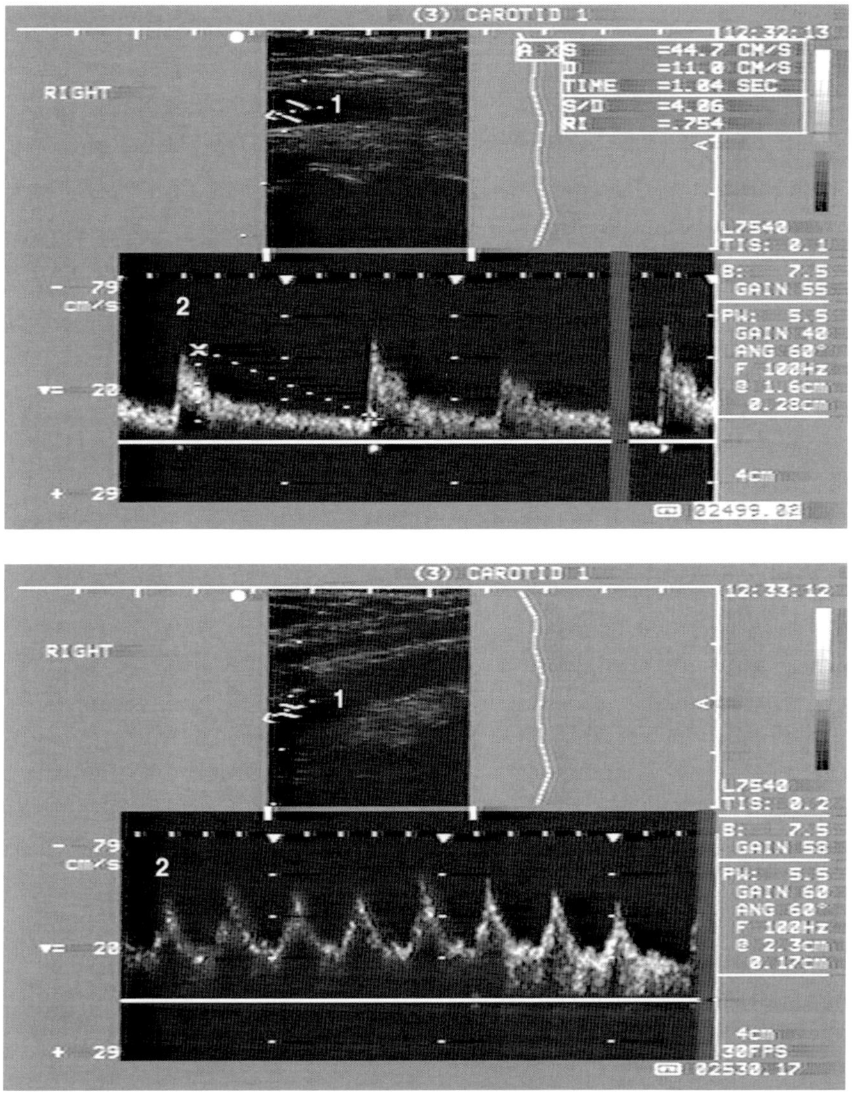

FIGURE 7.10. A: Duplex ultrasonography with Doppler spectral analysis of the right carotid system demonstrating the basal heart rate. *1*, Doppler sample was placed in the right internal carotid artery; *2*, Doppler spectrum shows basal heart rate. **B:** Duplex ultrasonography with Doppler spectral analysis demonstrating paroxysmal tachycardia after stimulation of the right carotid sinus by the transducer during the performance of carotid duplex sonography. *1*, Doppler sample was placed in the right internal carotid artery; *2*, Doppler spectrum shows paroxysmal tachycardia.

Diagnosis: Paradoxical response to carotid sinus stimulation. The normal physiologic response of baroreceptors in the wall of the carotid sinus to activation by stretching or deformation of the wall, is an increase of the vagal activity and a decrease of the sympathetic activity. A paroxysmal tachycardia developed in this patient after the stimulation of each carotid sinus by the transducer during the performance of carotid duplex ultrasonography. The patient was being given a calcium channel antagonist and digitalis to control the ventricular response to intermittent atrial fibrillation. Interaction between the carotid sinus baroreceptor response and these medications may explain this paradoxical response (9).

PEARLS AND PITFALLS

Pearls

- The bisferious pulse has two systolic peaks and either the first or the second peak may be the highest.
- The etiology of the bisferious pulse may be based on the highest peak.
- Pulsus alternans is defined as an alternating pulse pattern in which the beats occur at constant intervals but with regular alternation of the amplitude.
- The pattern of a bigeminal pulse is a regular coupling of two beats in rapid succession followed by a longer interval between a pair of beats than between the coupled beats themselves.

Pitfalls

- It is necessary to take into account the feature of the two systolic peaks of the bisferious pulse to avoid a misdiagnosis of hypertrophic cardiomyopathy as mixed aortic stenosis.
- The misinterpretation of pulsus alternans as bigeminal pulsus is avoided by the regular rhythm of the heart contracting.
- A compensatory pause is present after atrial premature beats, as well as after ventricular premature beats and can be misidentified by palpation.
- A characteristic feature of hypertrophic cardiomyopathy, both obstructive and nonobstructive, is a bisferious pulse.

QUESTIONS

1. Which of the following statements is true of the bisferious pulse?
   a. The bisferious pulse is a pulse with two systolic peaks.
   b. Either the first or the second peak may be the highest.
   c. Differentiation based on this criterion may help to discern the etiology of the pulse.
   d. All of the above
   e. None of the above

2. In the bisferious pulse of the hypertrophic cardiomyopathy, the initial systolic wave is wider and of greater amplitude.
   True or false?

3. In patients with hypertrophic obstructive cardiomyopathy (HOCM),
   a. the midsystolic dipping is not a characteristic for HOCM.
   b. it is called Brockenbrough phenomenon.
   c. an increased contractility will also increase the ventricular outflow.
   d. All of the above
   e. None of the above

4. In the combined lesion—stenosis and incompetence—of the aortic valve, the first systolic peak is always lower than the second.
   True or false?

5. The pattern of the bigeminal pulse shows a regular coupling of two beats with the interval between the pair of beats being ________ the interval between the coupled beats themselves.
   a. greater than
   b. shorter than
   c. equal to
   d. double
   e. half

6. In atrial fibrillation, the sequential pulses are ________ the same.
   a. always
   b. never
   c. sometimes
   d. usually
   e. rarely

7. Abnormalities of the sinus node function are rare in patients
   a. with atrial septal defect.
   b. after surgery.
   c. who use calcium channel blockers.
   d. All of the above
   e. None of the above

8. A full compensatory pause indicates that the interval between the normal beat immediately before and immediately after the ventricular premature beat is exactly twice the basal interval.
   True or false?

9. Which of the following statements is true of ectopic beats?
   a. They are often premature.
   b. Atrial (APBs), atrioventricular (JPBs), or ventricular (VPBs) premature beats may be found.
   c. APBs and VPBs are usually followed by a pause before the next normal beat.
   d. All of the above
   e. None of the above

10. Carotid sinus hypersensitivity
   a. can cause stroke.
   b. can appear after carotid sinus stimulation.
   c. can display abnormal carotid artery wall motion.
   d. All of the above
   e. None of the above

11. The normal physiologic response after activation of the baroreceptors in the wall of the carotid sinus is
   a. a decrease in vagal activity.
   b. an increase in vagal activity.
   c. a decrease in sympathetic activity.
   d. a and c
   e. b and c

12. The baroreceptors of the wall of the carotid sinus are the only baroreceptors that can be stimulated from the outside of the body.
   True or false?

13. The angulation of the right internal carotid artery revealed with color flow imaging in Figure 7.11
   a. is a tortuosity.
   b. corresponds to the grade I of Metz's classification of angulations of the internal carotid artery.
   c. corresponds to a kink of the internal carotid artery.
   d. a and b
   e. b and c

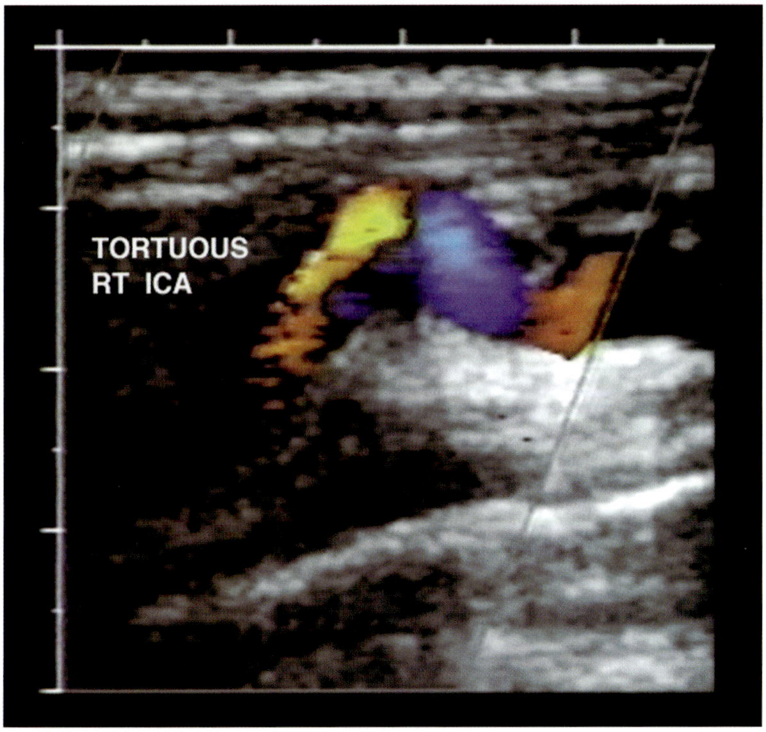

FIGURE 7.11. Right internal carotid artery. Lateral view. Longitudinal. Color.

Answers: **1.** d; **2.** True; **3.** b; **4.** True; **5.** a; **6.** b; **7.** e; **8.** True; **9.** d; **10.** d; **11.** e; **12.** True; **13.** d.

REFERENCES

1. Craige E, Smith D. Heart sounds: phonocardiography; carotid, apex, and jugular venous pulse tracings and systolic time intervals. In: Braunwald E, ed. *Heart disease,* 3rd ed. Philadelphia: WB Saunders, 1988.
2. Nesje OA, Enge I. External carotid pulse recordings in hypertrophic obstructive cardiomyopathy. *Acta Med Scand* 1977;202:197–202.
3. O'Rourke MF, Kelly R, Avolio A. The arterial pulse. Philadelphia: Lea & Febiger, 1982.
4. Feinstein AR, Hochstein E, Luisada A, et al. Glossary of cardiology in terms related to physical diagnosis: part IV. Arterial pulses. *Am J Cardiol* 1971;27:708–709.
5. Bigger JT Jr. The electrical activity of the heart. In: Schlant RC, Alexander RW, eds. *Hurst. The heart. Arteries and veins.* McGraw-Hill, 1994.
6. Carrasco HA, Fuenmayor A, Barboza J, et al. Effect of verapamil on normal sino-atrial node dysfunction and on sick sinus syndrome. *Am Heart J* 1978;96:760–771.
7. Goldberger AL, Goldberger E. *Clinical electrocardiography. A simplified approach,* 5th ed. St. Louis: Mosby, 1994.
8. Alayon A. Carotid artery wall motion correlates with carotid sinus hypersensitivity. Abstract presented at the proceedings of the 20th Annual Meeting of the American Society of Neuroimaging. San Juan, Puerto Rico, March 5–8, 1997.
9. Copen DL, Cirillo DP, Vassalle M. Tachycardia following vagal stimulation. *Am J Physiol* 1968;15:696–793.

CHAPTER 8

NORMAL VERTEBRAL ARTERY HEMODYNAMICS AND PATHOLOGY

The extracranial portion of the vertebral artery can be examined with duplex sonography. Because it is less anatomically accessible to the ultrasound probe, color-coded Doppler imaging is especially useful in examining the vertebral arteries. The principles underlying interpretation are similar to those for carotid duplex sonography, but the detection and classification of stenosis of vertebral artery by pulsed-wave Doppler criteria is more difficult than in the carotid system.

Systematic duplex examination of the vertebral artery segments includes the display of the ostium and pretransverse course, the intertransverse segments, and the atlas loop of the vertebral artery.

The vertebral arteries are deeply placed in the neck and, in the midcervical course, they are largely obscured by the acoustic shadowing resulting from the transverse processes of the cervical vertebrae as they pass through them, from C6 to C2. For this reason, Doppler vertebral examination is subject to difficulties and limitations not encountered in other cervical vessels.

Continuous wave Doppler sonography was initially the most important tool for noninvasive investigation of the extracranial vertebral arteries. The Doppler spectrum recorded from an intertransverse segment of a normal vertebral artery demonstrates a high diastolic flow velocity and low pulsatility, indicating low vascular resistance in the territory of supply. Doppler criteria and their relationship to a grade of stenosis of the vertebral artery have been difficult to define because of the small diameter of the artery and anatomic variations.

The introduction of color-coded Doppler sonography facilitates the identification of the ostium and proximal segment of the vertebral artery, which is the predominant location of extracranial vertebral stenosis.

The following cases demonstrate the examination technique of the vertebral arteries, which includes B-mode imaging, Doppler spectrum analysis, and color-coded Doppler sonography. Findings associated with normal and various pathologic conditions as a basis for diagnosis and basic clinical studies are described.

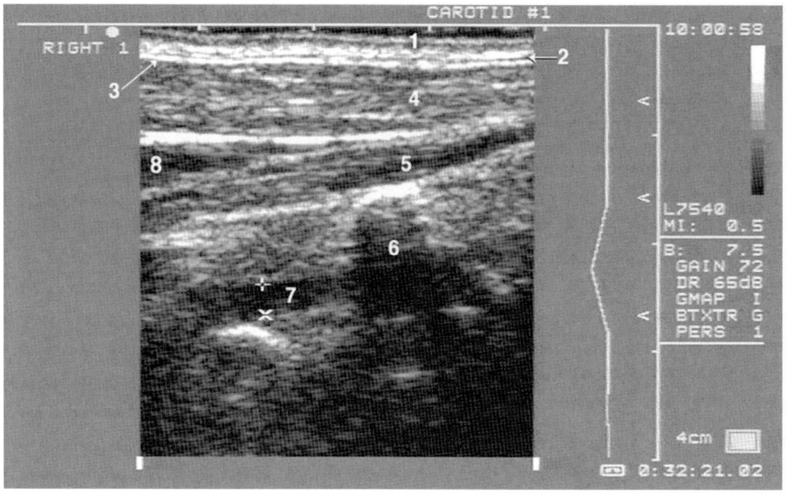

FIGURE 8.1. Right vertebral artery. Anteroposterior view. Longitudinal. Gray scale. *1*, Skin and superficial cervical fascia; *2*, platysma; *3*, deep cervical fascia; *4*, sternocleidomastoid muscle; *5*, right common carotid artery; *6*, acoustic shadowing (transverse process); *7*, right vertebral artery; *8*, right internal jugular vein.

Diagnosis: Vertebral artery. Normal anatomy. The vertebral artery arises from the superoposterior aspect of the subclavian, passes through the foramina of all cervical transverse processes except the seventh, and enters the cranium via the foramen magnum. The first part ascends posteriorly between the longus colli and scalenus anterior, posterior to the common carotid artery and posterior to the seventh cervical transverse process. The second part ascends through the transverse foramina, vertically to the transverse process of the axis through which it turns laterally to the transverse foramen. The third part lies medial to the rectus capitis lateralis, curving back behind the lateral mass and then in a groove on the upper surface of the posterior arch of the atlas, entering the vertebral canal below the inferior border of the posterior atlantooccipital membrane (1).

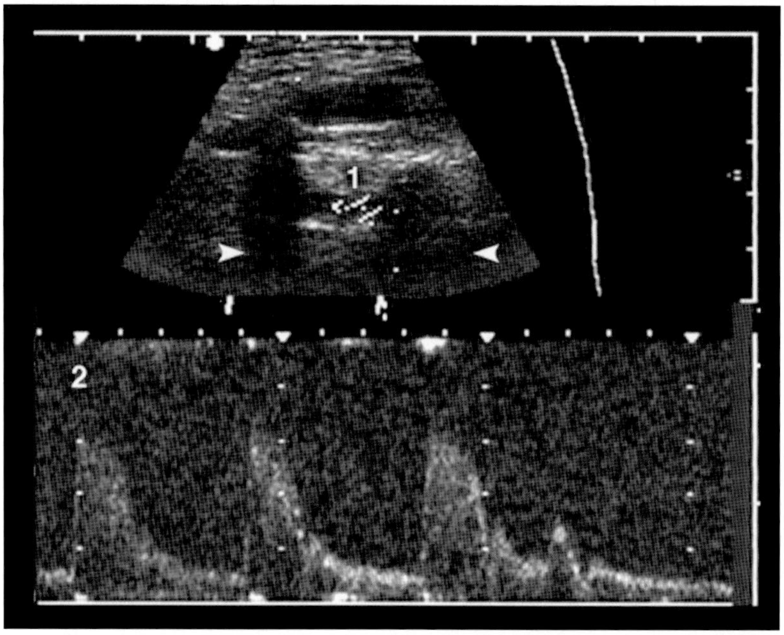

FIGURE 8.2. Vertebral artery. *1*, Sample volume placed at the vertebral artery; *2*, Doppler spectrum of the vertebral artery; acoustic shadowing resulting from the transverse process of the vertebra.

Diagnosis: Vertebral artery identification. To identify the vertebral artery, start with a longitudinal view of the carotid artery, approximately midway between the clavicle and mandible. Then shift the image plane laterally until shadows of the transverse processes of the cervical vertebrae are identified. The vertebral arteries are seen between the transverse processes (2).

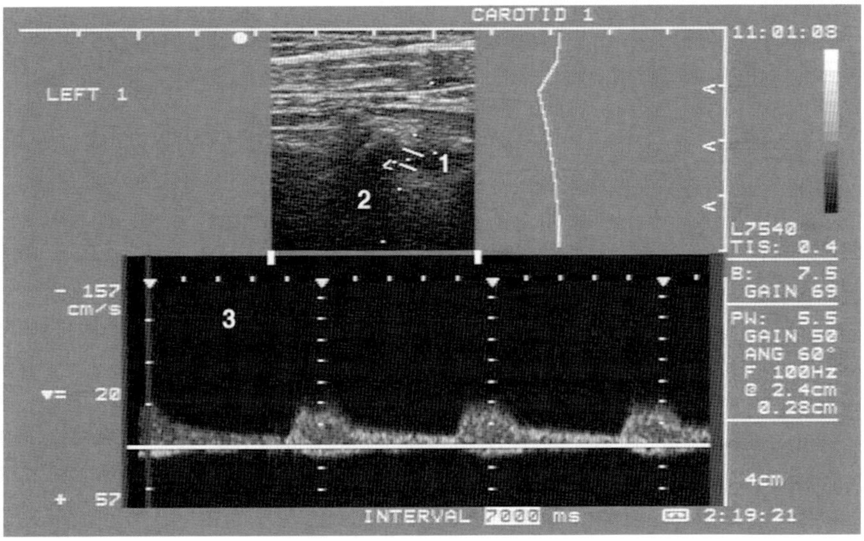

FIGURE 8.3. Left vertebral artery. Anteroposterior view. Longitudinal. Gray scale. Doppler spectrum. *1*, Doppler sample gate placed in the left vertebral artery; *2*, acoustic shadowing resulting from transverse process of the vertebra; *3*, normal Doppler waveform of the vertebral artery.

Diagnosis: Vertebral artery, normal Doppler spectrum. The V1 (pretransverse) segment and V2 (transverse) segment of the vertebral artery can be imaged by moving the transducer cephalad in the anteroposterior plane. The V3 segment as well as V4 or intracranial course of the vertebral can be imaged by means of color Doppler imaging alone. After imaging vertebral arteries in the different segments, spectral analysis of the blood flow and velocity measurements can be performed. The velocity spectral waveform of the vertebral flow shows a typical low-resistance pattern. Regularly spaced areas of acoustic shadowing resulting from the transverse processes of the vertebrae and the vessel lumens between them can be identified (3).

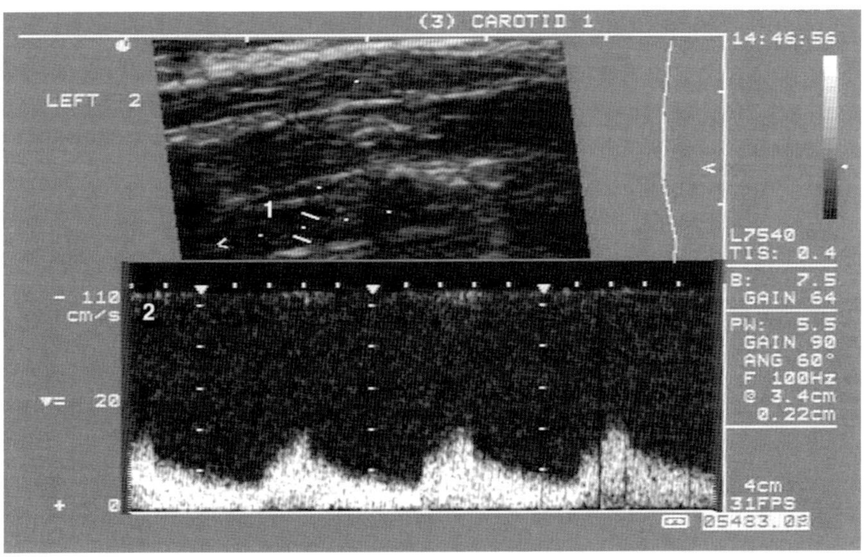

FIGURE 8.4. Left vertebral artery. Anteroposterior view. Longitudinal. Gray scale. Doppler spectrum. *1*, Sample volume placed in the left vertebral artery; *2*, Doppler waveform shows typical poststenotic waveform.

Diagnosis: Vertebral artery stenosis. The origin of the vertebral artery is the second most common stenosis site of the cervical vessels. Because of technical problems in placing the sample volume in the narrowest part of the stenosis, there are insufficient data concerning the relationship between the flow velocity and the grade of stenosis at the origin of the vertebral artery. In clinical practice, the indirect signs are important, especially when the origin of the vertebral artery cannot be visualized. A proximally located severe stenosis can be presumed based on decreases in pulsatility and systolic and diastolic velocities (4).

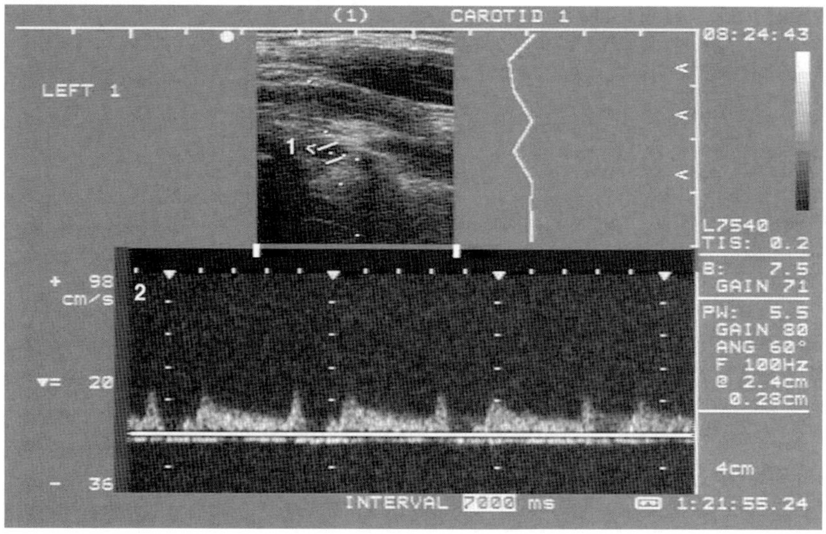

FIGURE 8.5. Left vertebral artery. Anteroposterior view. Longitudinal. Gray scale. Doppler spectrum. *1,* Sample placed in the left vertebral artery; *2,* Doppler spectrum shows systolic deceleration.

Diagnosis: Subclavian steal syndrome. Systolic deceleration in the vertebral artery. The subclavian steal syndrome can result from stenosis or occlusion of the subclavian artery or brachiocephalic trunk proximal to the origin of the ipsilateral vertebral artery. The changes in the blood flow in the vertebral artery depend on the grade of stenosis of the subclavian artery, resulting in an incomplete or complete steal effect. In cases of moderate stenosis, only a systolic deceleration of the flow velocity can be observed. The systolic deceleration appears as a small notch commencing shortly before the systolic peak. The low point of the notch coincides with the systolic peak of the freely perfused vertebral artery (5).

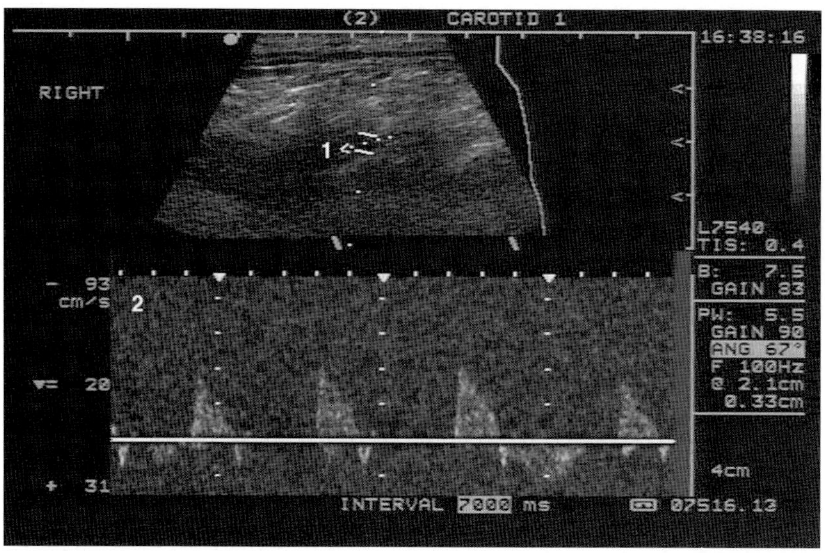

FIGURE 8.6. Right vertebral artery. Anteroposterior view. Longitudinal. Gray scale. Doppler spectrum. *1,* Sample volume placed in the right vertebral artery; *2,* Doppler spectrum of the right vertebral artery shows alternating flow.

Diagnosis: Subclavian steal syndrome. Alternating flow in the vertebral artery. In high-grade stenosis of the subclavian artery, the flow becomes alternating directly toward the arm in systole and toward the brain in diastole. This change of flow direction in the vertebral artery is cardiac phase-dependent. An increase of flow velocity in the antegrade direction is seen at the start of the systolic wave. Alternating flow has the positive effect of protecting the vessel from stasis and thrombus formation (6).

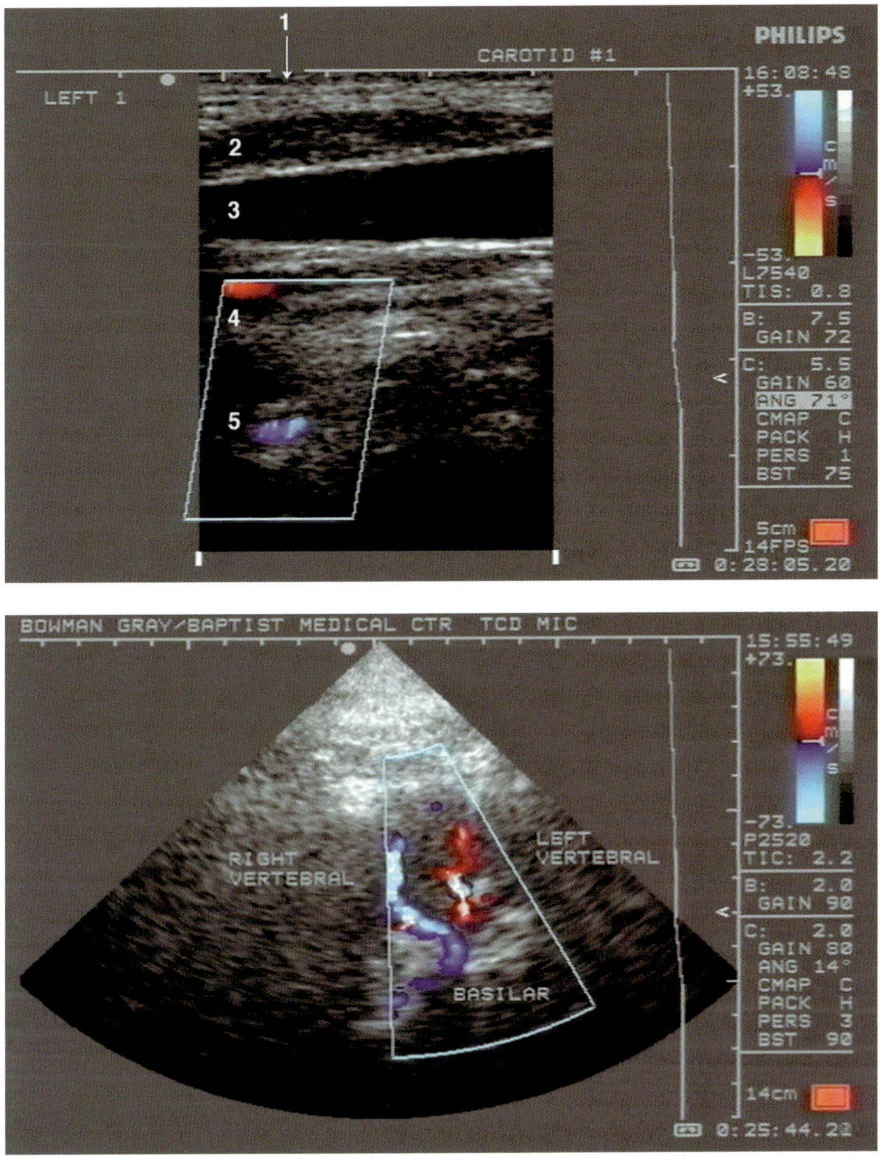

A

B

FIGURE 8.7. A: Left vertebral artery. Anteroposterior view. Longitudinal. Color flow imaging. *1*, Skin, superficial cervical fascia and platysma; *2*, sternocleidomastoid muscle; *3*, left internal jugular vein; *4*, left common carotid artery, antegrade flow *(red)*; *5*, left vertebral artery, retrograde flow *(blue)*. **B:** Transcranial color-coded duplex. Transforaminal approach. Right vertebral artery, antegrade flow, *blue*; left vertebral artery, retrograde flow, *red*; basilar artery, antegrade flow, *blue*.

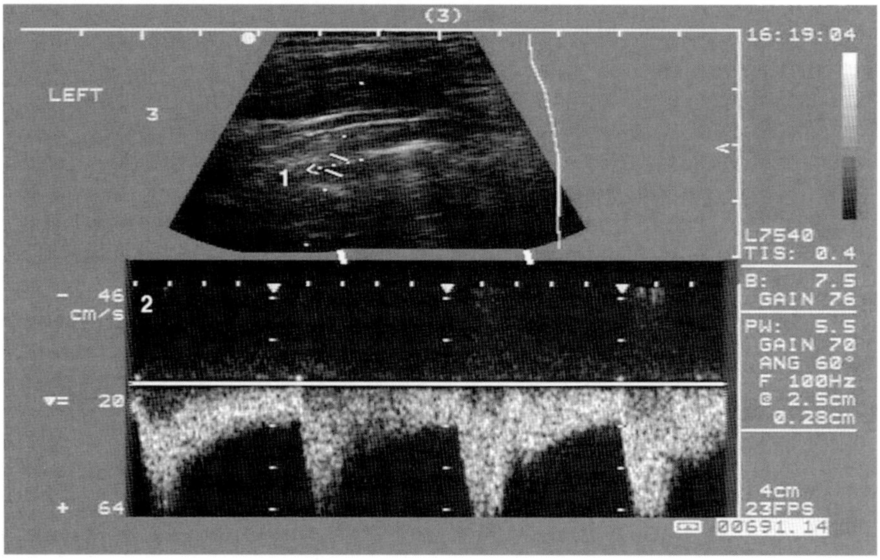

FIGURE 8.8. Left vertebral artery. Anteroposterior view. Longitudinal. Gray scale. Doppler spectrum. *1*, Sample volume placed in the left vertebral artery; Doppler spectrum shows reversed flow in the left vertebral artery.

Diagnosis: Subclavian steal syndrome. Retrograde flow in the vertebral artery. The retrograde flow down the left vertebral artery throughout the cardiac cycle reflects a complete steal effect resulting from a high-grade stenosis or occlusion of the ipsilateral, proximal subclavian artery. In this situation, the subclavian artery is supplied by the retrograde vertebral artery, and the waveform is similar to that of the subclavian artery (7).

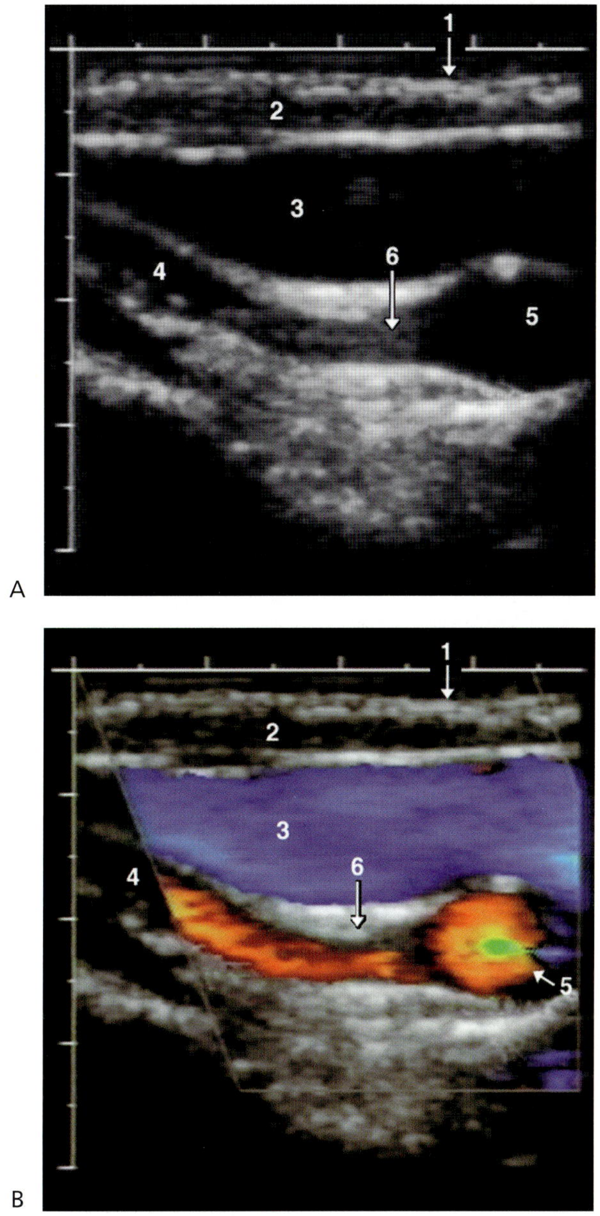

FIGURE 8.9. Right vertebral artery. Lateral view. Longitudinal. Gray scale **(A)** and color **(B)**. *1*, Skin and superficial cervical fascia; *2*, sternocleidomastoid muscle; *3*, internal jugular vein; *4*, right vertebral artery; *5*, right subclavian artery; *6*, low-echogenicity plaque at the origin of the right vertebral artery.

Diagnosis: Low-echoic plaque at the origin of the right vertebral artery. Atherosclerotic stenosis or occlusion occurs primarily at the vertebral artery origin. The second most common site of atherosclerotic obstruction is intracranial, just beyond the C1 vertebral arch. Less commonly, plaque develops more diffusely at the vertebral transverse foramina, in the intracranial segments, or in the intracranial branches. Because most plaques occurring in the vertebral arteries are fibrous rather than fatty, vertebrobasilar insufficiency symptoms are usually not attributable to embolization. High-grade stenosis is readily identified by color-coded duplex sonography because of the visible reduction in diameter and direct visualization of hemodynamic abnormalities. High-resolution sonography is also often able to detect atheromatous lesions of the proximal vertebral artery, even in the absence of significant stenosis. The ability to analyze the surface and structural characteristics of the plaque is of importance in identifying potential sources of local embolism (8).

PEARLS AND PITFALLS

Pearls

- The vertebral artery arises from the superoposterior aspect of the subclavian artery and passes through the foramina of the cervical transverse processes.
- The origin of vertebral artery is the second most common stenosis site of the cervical vessels and pathologic studies. Because of technical problems in placing the sample, there are insufficient data regarding flow velocities and the grade of stenosis.
- The diagnosis of vertebral artery stenosis in clinical practice is based on indirect signs with decreases in pulsatility and systolic and diastolic velocities.
- The velocity spectral waveform of vertebral flow shows a typical low-resistance pattern.

Pitfalls

- In complete subclavian steal syndrome, the subclavian artery is supplied by the retrograde flow from the vertebral artery and the waveform of the vertebral artery can be misrecognized as the subclavian artery.
- Continuous examination of the vertebral arteries is not possible because of the transverse processes of the cervical vertebrae.
- It is difficult to obtain optimal angles for Doppler insonation at the origin of the vertebral artery, making velocity measurements less accurate.
- The diagnosis of vertebral artery occlusion is difficult to make.

QUESTIONS

1. The Doppler sample (Fig. 8.10) was placed in the left vertebral artery. The first Doppler waveform was obtained during the compression test of the left upper arm; afterward, the cuff was released (*arrowhead*) and the baseline Doppler waveform appeared. This Doppler pattern corresponds to which of the following?
   a. A "stolen" pattern waveform from the vertebral artery supplies the underperfused arm.
   b. During the compression test, the flow direction in the vertebral artery was antegrade.
   c. Stenosis of the origin of the subclavian artery can be suspected.
   d. All of the above
   e. None of the above

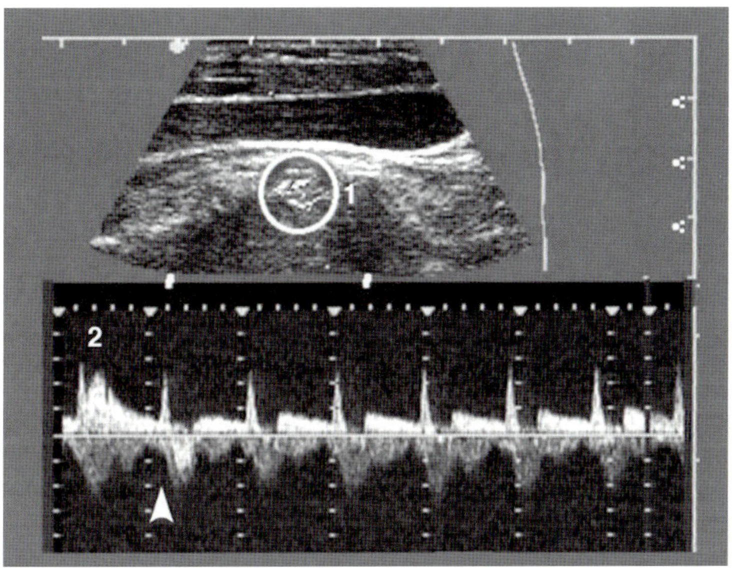

FIGURE 8.10. Left vertebral artery. Lateral view. Longitudinal. Gray scale. Doppler spectrum.

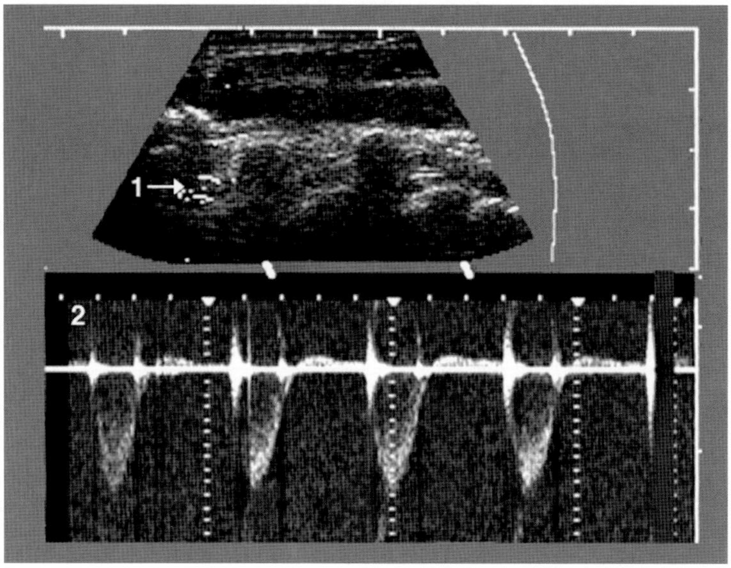

FIGURE 8.11. Left vertebral artery. Lateral view. Longitudinal. Gray scale. Doppler spectrum. *1*, Sample volume placed in the left vertebral artery; *2*, Doppler spectrum of the left vertebral artery.

2. The Doppler spectrum shown in Figure 8.11 corresponds with a vertebral steal because there is total occlusion of the left brachiocephalic trunk.
   True or false?

3. In the normal anatomy of the vertebral artery,
   a. the artery arises from the superior aspect of the aortic arch on the left side.
   b. the artery passes anterior to the foramina of all cervical transverse processes.
   c. the artery is posterior to the common carotid artery.
   d. All of the above
   e. None of the above

4. In vertebral artery stenosis,
   a. it is uncommon for the stenosis to be at the origin of the vertebral artery.
   b. it is very easy to know the grade of the stenosis by placing the sample volume in the narrowest part of the stenosis.
   c. indirect signs are important in clinical practice for diagnosis of stenosis at the origin of the vertebral artery.
   d. All of the above
   e. None of the above

5. The origin of the vertebral artery is the second most common stenosis site of the cervical vessels.
   True or false?

6. The subclavian steal syndrome can result from stenosis or occlusion of the ________ distal to the origin of the ipsilateral vertebral artery.
   a. subclavian artery
   b. brachiocephalic trunk
   c. ascending aorta
   d. All of the above
   e. None of the above

7. In subclavian steal syndrome,
   a. the changes in the blood flow in the vertebral artery depend on the grade of stenosis of the subclavian artery.
   b. the changes in the blood flow in the vertebral artery depend on the grade of stenosis of the brachiocephalic artery.
   c. in cases of moderate stenosis, only a systolic deceleration of the flow velocity can be observed.
   d. All of the above
   e. None of the above

8. In high-grade stenosis of the subclavian artery with subclavian steal syndrome, the flow becomes alternating directly toward the arm in systole and toward the brain in diastole.
   True or false?

9. In subclavian steal syndrome, the flow in the ipsilateral vertebral artery
   a. becomes alternating in high-grade stenosis of the subclavian artery.
   b. changes in flow direction and is cardiac phase-dependent.
   c. the alternating flow protects the vessel from thrombus formation.
   d. All of the above
   e. None of the above

10. The retrograde flow down the vertebral artery throughout the cardiac cycle reflects a(n) ________ steal effect resulting from ________ of the ipsilateral subclavian artery.
   a. incomplete, occlusion
   b. incomplete, mild stenosis
   c. complete, occlusion
   d. complete, mild stenosis
   e. None of the above

11. The Doppler waveform in the vertebral artery in a complete subclavian steal syndrome is similar to the ipsilateral subclavian artery.
   True or false?

12. The vertebral arteries cannot be identified because of acoustic shadowing of the transverse process of the vertebra.
   True or false?

13. In relation to the vertebral artery,
    a. the vertebral Doppler spectrum shows a typical low-resistance pattern.
    b. the vessel lumen appears between the regularly spaced areas of acoustic shadowing as a result of the transverse processes of the vertebrae.
    c. its intracranial course can be imaged by means of the color Doppler imaging alone.
    d. All of the above
    e. None of the above

Answers: **1.** d; **2.** False; **3.** c; **4.** c; **5.** True; **6.** e; **7.** d; **8.** True; **9.** d; **10.** c; **11.** True; **12.** False; **13.** d.

REFERENCES

1. Williams PL. *Gray's anatomy. The anatomical basis of medicine and surgery,* 38th ed. New York: Churchill-Livingstone, 1995.
2. Bartels E. Vertebral sonography. In: Tegeler CH, Babikian VL, Gomez CR, eds. *Neurosonology.* Chicago: Mosby–Year Book, 1996.
3. Rae RE. Cerebrovascular sonography, Doppler and noninvasive examinations. In: *Textbook of diagnostic ultrasonography,* 4th ed. St. Louis: Mosby, 1995.
4. Moosy J. Morphology, sites and epidemiology of cerebral atherosclerosis. In: Milliken C, ed. *Cerebrovascular disease.* Baltimore: Williams & Wilkins, 1986.
5. von Reutern G, Budingen HJ, Freund HJ. Doppler-sonographische diagnostik von stenosen und verschlussen der vertebralarterien und des subclaviansteal-syndromes. *Arch Psychiat Nervenkr* 1976;222:209–222.
6. Klingelhofer J, Conrad B, Benecke R, et al. Transcranial Doppler ultrasonography of carotid-basilar collateral circulation in subclavian steal. *Stroke* 1988;19:1036–1042.
7. von Reutern GM, von Budingen HJ. *Ultrasound diagnosis of cerebrovascular disease. Doppler sonography of the extra- and intracranial arteries. Duplex scanning.* Stuttgart, Germany: Georg Thieme Verlag, 1993.
8. Moossy J. Morphology, sites and epidemiology of cerebral atherosclerosis. In: Millikan CH, ed. *Cerebrovascular disease.* Baltimore: Williams & Wilkins.

CHAPTER 9

NORMAL INTERNAL JUGULAR VEIN AND INCOMPETENT VALVES

The cervical veins can be divided into superficial and deep veins with respect to their position relative to the cervical fascia. The largest vein in the neck, the internal jugular vein, is easily assessed sonographically. It descends lateral to the internal and common carotid arteries to its junction with the brachiocephalic vein.

A valve can be seen in the inferior bulb area. This is the only valve between the right atrium of the heart and the brain.

The importance of the internal jugular vein has been underestimated. The competency of the valve can avoid the reverse flow of venous blood during Valsalva maneuver or during sudden increases in intrathoracic pressure. This might lead to intracranial venous engorgement and increased intracranial pressure with possible medullary compression.

For the examination of the internal jugular vein, the head is rotated slightly back and to the opposite side. The internal jugular vein is easily found lateral to the carotid artery and all parts of the vein must be examined in longitudinal and transverse planes. In contrast to the arteries, veins have a thin, highly echogenic wall without layers. The competence of the jugular valve must be done with pulsed Doppler techniques during Valsalva maneuver.

Color-coded Doppler sonography of the internal jugular vein allows observation of its cyclic flow velocity changes in real time and it plays a role in the indirect diagnosis of pathologic conditions.

The cases focus on the examination technique, normal appearance of the vein, and pathologic findings, including the presence of spontaneous echo contrast and jugular valve incompetence.

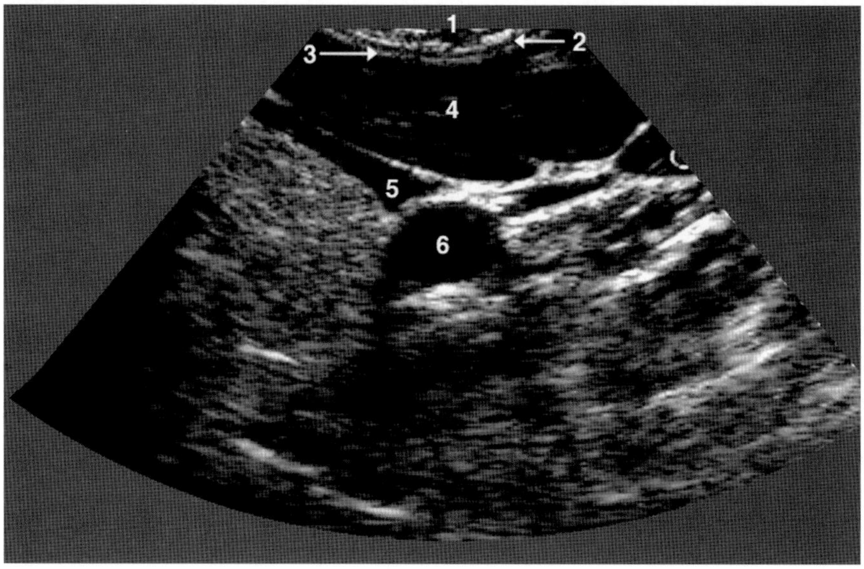

FIGURE 9.1. Right common carotid artery. Transverse view. Gray scale. *1*, Skin and superficial cervical fascial; *2*, platysma; *3*, deep cervical fascia; *4*, sternocleidomastoid muscle; *5*, internal jugular vein; *6*, common carotid artery.

Diagnosis: Differentiation between the carotid artery and jugular vein. The common carotid artery lies adjacent to the jugular vein; however, the two vessels can be differentiated. The carotid artery exhibits a pulsatile flow pattern, while the jugular vein has a continuous or undulating low-velocity signal. The caliber of the carotid arteries is fairly constant, whereas the caliber of the jugular vein varies in response to respiration and pressure of the transducer. The carotid artery is thick-walled with specular reflection of the intima, which is not seen at the jugular vein wall (1).

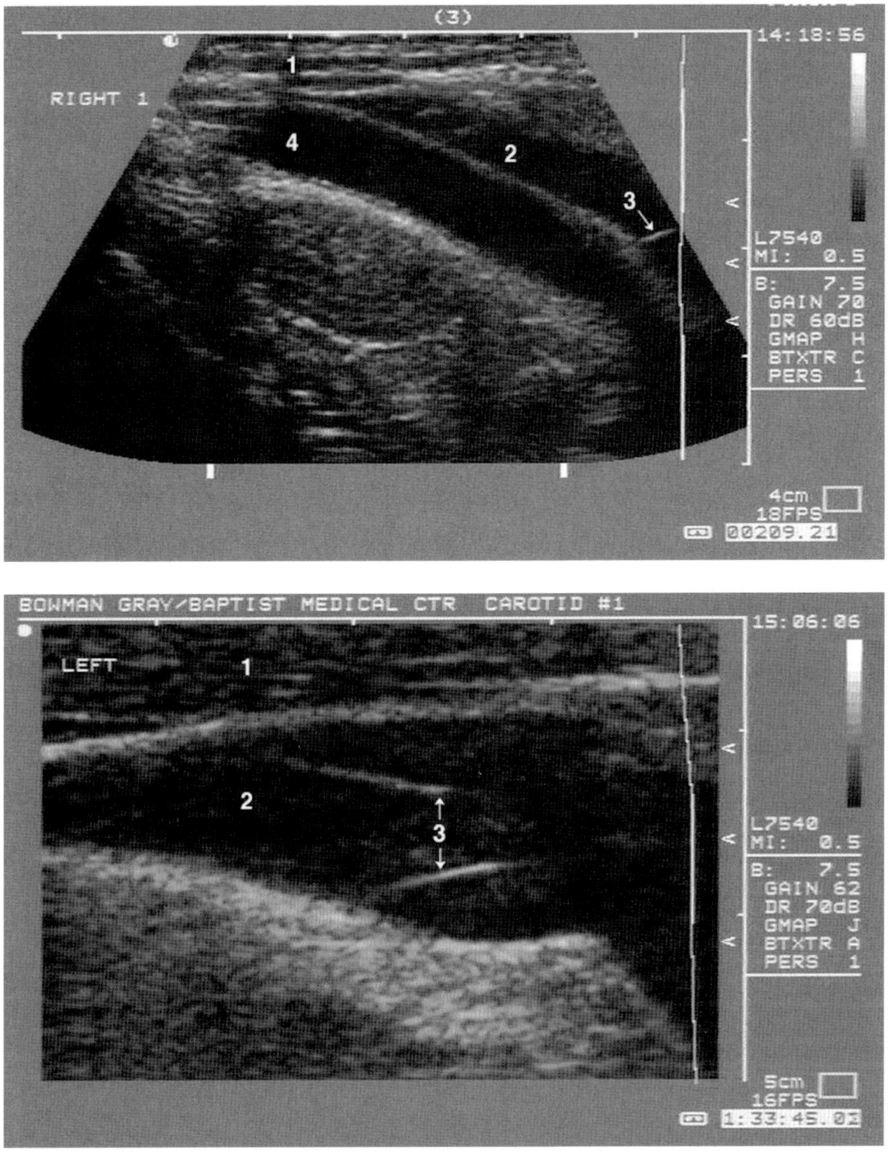

A

B

FIGURE 9.2. A: Right common carotid artery and jugular vein. Anteroposterior view. Longitudinal. Gray scale. *1,* Sternocleidomastoid muscle; *2,* right internal jugular vein; *3,* jugular valve; *4,* right common carotid artery. **B:** Left internal jugular vein. Anteroposterior view. Longitudinal. Gray scale. *1,* Sternocleidomastoid muscle; *2,* left internal jugular vein; *3,* valve leaflets.

Diagnosis: Internal jugular vein and jugular valve. Normal anatomy. This large vein collects blood from the skull, brain, superficial parts of the face, and much of the neck. It begins at the cranial base in the posterior compartment of the jugular foramen, continuous with the sigmoid sinus. At its origin is the superior bulb, lying inferior to the posterior part of the tympanic floor. The vein descends in the carotid sheath, to join with the subclavian vein to form the brachiocephalic vein. It is also dilated near its end as its inferior bulb, above which it contains venous valves that may be one, two, three, or four cusps. The most common is bicuspid. Sonographically, the internal jugular vein presents as an easily compressible vessel adjacent to the internal carotid artery at its dorsolateral aspect and follows the common carotid artery laterally. When imaging is performed in an anteroposterior view and on longitudinal section, both the anterior and posterior wall can be identified (2).

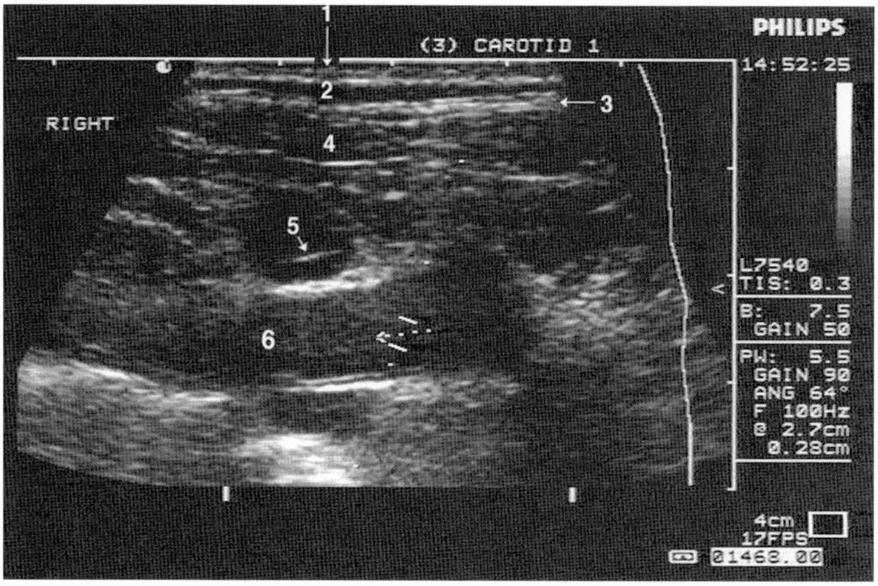

A

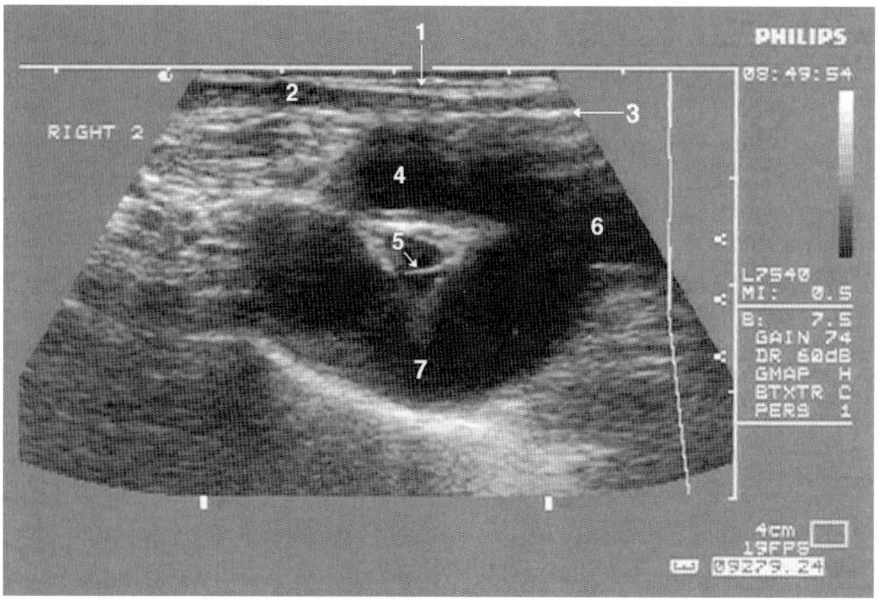

B

FIGURE 9.3. A: Right internal jugular vein. Transverse view. Gray scale. Supraclavicular approach. *1*, Skin and superficial cervical fascia; *2*, platysma; *3*, deep cervical fascia; *4*, sternocleidomastoid muscle; *5*, right internal jugular vein and valve cusp; *6*, right subclavian artery. **B:** Right internal jugular vein and brachiocephalic trunk. Transverse view. Gray scale. Supraclavicular approach. *1*, Skin and superficial cervical fascia; *2*, platysma; *3*, deep cervical fascia; *4*, right common carotid artery; *5*, right internal jugular vein and jugular valve; *6*, innominate artery; *7*, right subclavian artery.

Diagnosis: Internal jugular vein and jugular valves. Normal anatomy. The anatomic relations at the level of the inferior bulb of the internal jugular vein are posterior, medial, and superficially. Posterior to the vein are the scalenus anterior, thyrocervical trunk, vertebral vein, and first part of the subclavian artery. On the left side, it also crosses anterior to the thoracic duct. Medial to the vein are the internal and common carotid arteries, and the vagus nerve lies between vein and arteries. Superficially, the vein is overlapped by the sternocleidomastoid muscle (3).

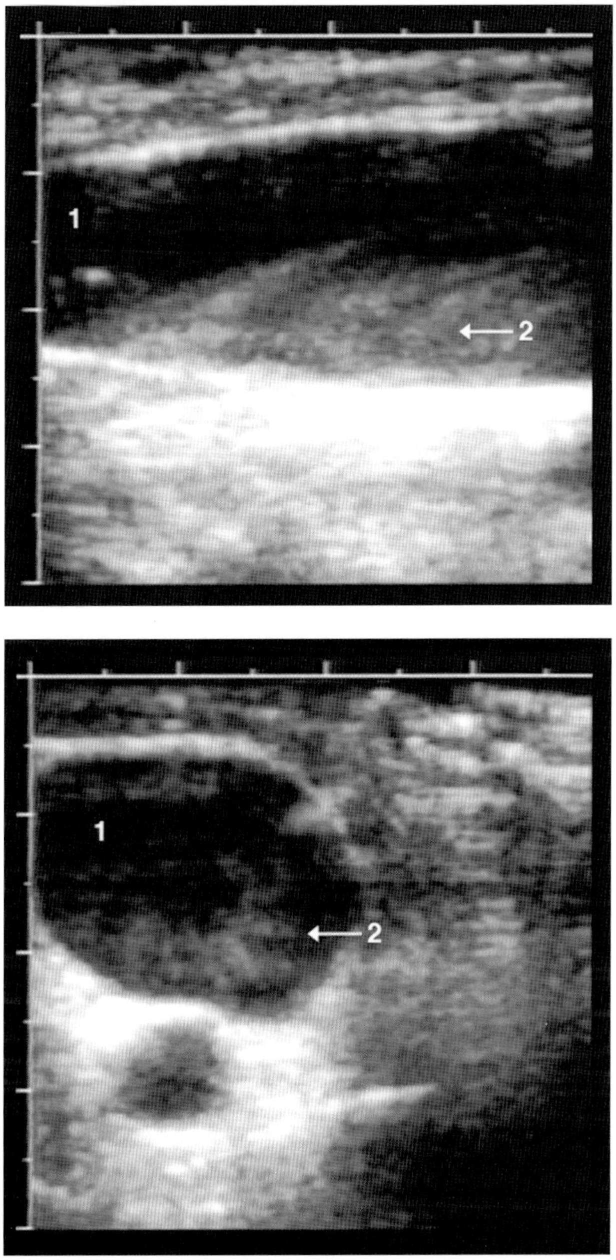

FIGURE 9.4. Right internal jugular vein. Lateral view. Gray scale. Longitudinal **(A)** and transverse **(B)**. *1*, Right internal jugular vein; *2*, spontaneous echo contrast in the internal jugular vein.

Diagnosis: Spontaneous echo contrast in the internal jugular vein. Whether the existence of spontaneous echo contrast (SEC) in venous blood does or does not represent a pathologic process is uncertain. However, SEC in brachial vessels has been observed in patients with cardiovascular or cerebrovascular disease, diabetes, cancer and congestive heart failure. The cellular basis for SEC is thought to be either red cell aggregates, or platelet aggregates. Aspirin therapy would not be expected to modify SEC if it is derived from red cell aggregates, but could modify SEC if it is coming from platelet aggregates. After 7 days of treatment with aspirin, some authors have observed a progressive decline in the amount of spontaneous echo contrast in the brachial veins. These results indicate that a component of SEC responds to the administration of aspirin. This confirms the hypothesis that circulating platelet aggregates occur in humans. Additional studies are recommended to confirm if the SEC is a marker for the platelet activation which occurs with aging and other risk factors for atherosclerosis (4).

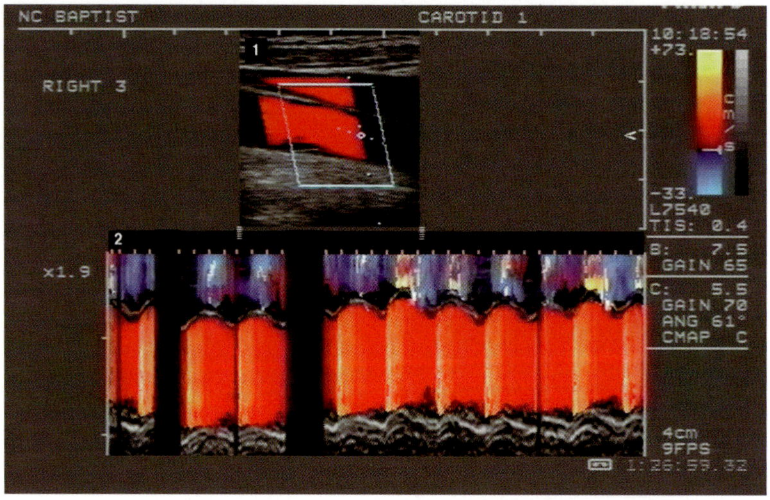

FIGURE 9.5. Right common carotid artery and internal jugular vein. Longitudinal view. Color. M-mode display. *1*, The red color in both, internal jugular vein *(above)* and right common carotid *(below)*, indicates the existence of reflux in the internal jugular vein; *2*, the M-mode display with color superimposed shows a reverse flow in the internal jugular vein *(red areas in the blue background, above)* during the cardiac cycle resulting from jugular valve incompetence, with normal antegrade flow in the common carotid artery *(red, below)*.

Diagnosis: Jugular valve incompetence. The jugular valve is the only valve between the right atrium of the heart and the brain. The clinical importance of the jugular valve has not been extensively studied and the incidence of its incompetency is not known. It has been implicated in tricuspid insufficiency, the respiratory brain syndrome, blood flow mechanics of cardiopulmonary resuscitation, and forward flow in sustained coughing. Although pulsed Doppler recordings can demonstrate valvular competency with the Valsalva maneuver, new studies have been done with color flow imaging (5).

PEARLS AND PITFALLS

Pearls

- The jugular valve is the only valve between the right atrium of the heart and the brain.
- The existence of spontaneous echo contrast in venous blood represents slow flow and possible other pathologies.
- The clinical importance of the jugular valve has not been extensively studied.
- The double arterial wall echoes seen on B-mode images because of specular reflection of the intima, are not seen at the jugular vein wall.

Pitfalls

- Turbulence related to flow deceleration in the widened lumen of the inferior bulb of the internal jugular vein is common, and without appropriate maneuver it can be misdiagnosed as jugular valve incompetence.
- With a high gain setting that is used in searching for a high-grade stenosis, the sample volume expands. This may lead to the reception of Doppler signals from the adjacent jugular vein, which can be misinterpreted as a Doppler signal originating from an occluded arterial segment.
- The marked widening of the jugular vein seen in B-mode image during Valsalva maneuver, can serve to avoid the misidentification of the jugular vein as the common carotid artery.
- Compression of the jugular vein by the probe can lead to reverberation artifacts. This can cause a misdiagnosis in the presence of a plaque in the near wall of the common carotid artery.

QUESTIONS

1. The internal jugular vein
   a. collects blood from the skull, brain, face and neck.
   b. begins at the cranial base in the posterior compartment of the jugular foramen.
   c. joins with the subclavian vein to form the brachiocephalic vein.
   d. All of the above
   e. None of the above
3. The jugular valve
   a. is the biggest valve between the right atrium of the heart and the brain.
   b. has been implicated in the respiratory brain death syndrome.
   c. has an incidence of incompetency of about 1%.
   d. All of the above
   e. None of the above
4. The valve of the right internal jugular vein (Fig. 9.6)
   a. has only one cusp.
   b. is bicuspid.
   c. is tricuspid.
   d. All of the above
   e. None of the above

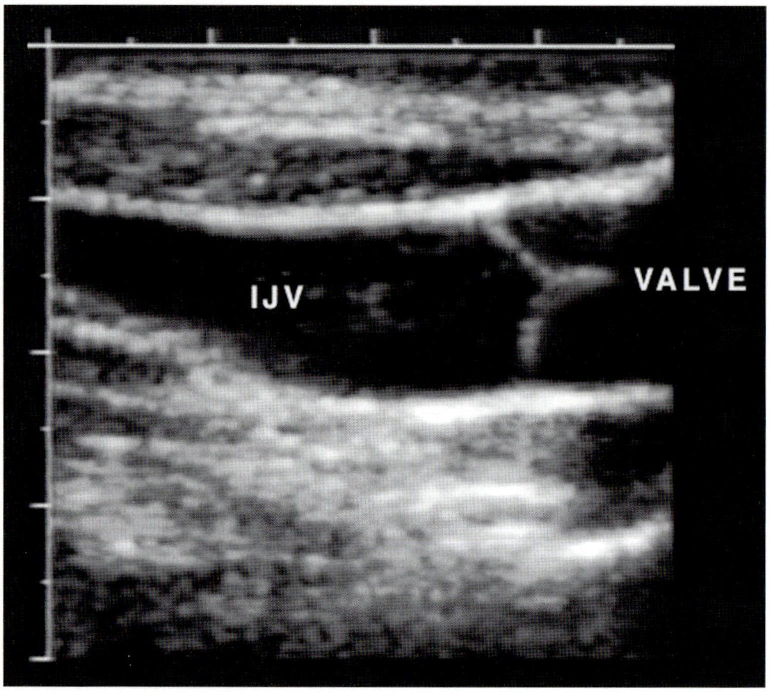

FIGURE 9.6. Diagnosis: Valve of the internal jugular vein. Right internal jugular vein (*IJV*). Lateral view. Longitudinal. Gray scale.

Answers: 1. d; 2. True; 3. c; 4. b.

REFERENCES

1. Zwiebel WJ. Color-duplex features of normal and abnormal carotid arteries. In: Zwiebel WJ, ed. *Introduction to vascular ultrasonography,* 3rd ed. Philadelphia: WB Saunders, 1992.
2. Muller HR. Ultrasonic imaging of the internal jugular vein. *J Neuroimaging* 1991;1: 74–78.
3. Williams PL. *Gray's anatomy. The anatomical basis of medicine and surgery,* 38th ed. New York: Churchill-Livingstone, 1995.
4. Kearney K, Mahony C. Effect of aspirin on spontaneous contrast in the brachial veins of normal subjects. *Am J Cardiol* 1995;75:924–928.
5. Brownlow RL Jr, McKinney WM. Ultrasonic evaluation of jugular venous valve competence. *J Ultrasound Med* 1985;4:169–172.

CHAPTER 10

ARTIFACT FACTS VERSUS ARTIFACTS

In sonography, an artifact is anything that is not properly indicative of the structures imaged and is caused by some characteristic of the imaging technique.

Some artifacts can lead to important errors in the interpretation of the image or display, but other artifacts are useful. This is because some ultrasound imaging artifacts provide valuable information on the nature of objects or lesions that might not be apparent with other imaging methods.

Artifacts in ultrasound imaging occur as structures that are not real, that are missing, that are improperly located; or have improper brightness, shape, or size.

Spectral artifact is an incorrect presentation of Doppler flow information. *Aliasing* is the most common artifact encountered in Doppler ultrasound and indicates the improper representation of information that has been insufficiently sampled.

Artifacts that occur with color flow imaging are color presentations of artifacts that are seen in gray-scale imaging and Doppler spectral displays. The original concept of color flow systems was that the direction of blood flow could be shown by the use of different colors, and a change in the velocity in either direction could be shown by the degree of saturation of the color.

Several ultrasound imaging, spectral, and color flow imaging artifacts are shown in this chapter. These help provide a proper understanding of artifacts and how to deal with them.

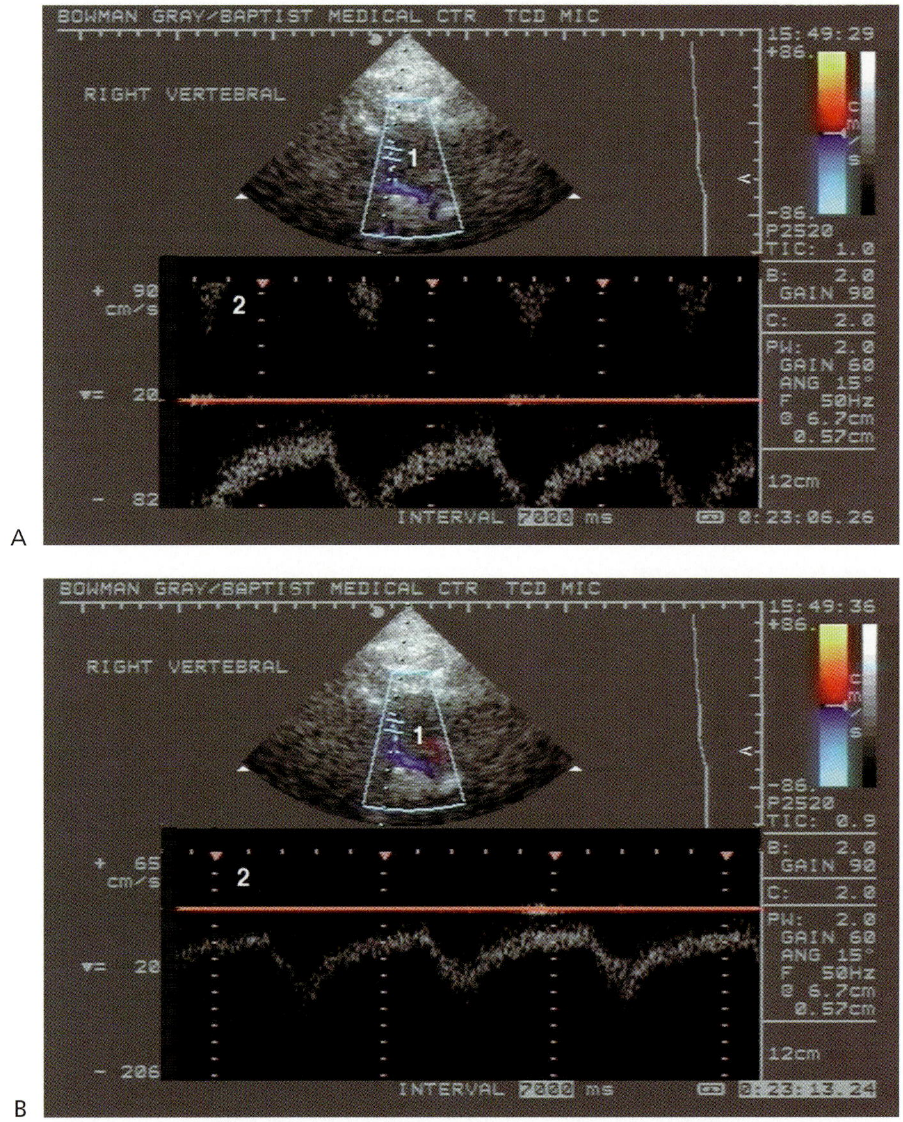

FIGURE 10.1. A: Transcranial color-coded duplex. Transforaminal approach. *1*, Doppler sample was placed in the right vertebral artery; *2*, Doppler spectrum shows aliasing. **B:** Transcranial color-coded duplex. Transforaminal approach. *1*, Doppler sample was placed in the right vertebral artery; *2*, Doppler spectrum was corrected by proper baseline shift.

Artifact: Aliasing. Aliasing is the most common artifact encountered in Doppler ultrasound. It indicates the improper representation of Doppler-shift information that has been insufficiently sampled. It occurs when the true Doppler shift exceeds one half of the pulse repetition frequency, which is the number of pulses (samples) per second (1).

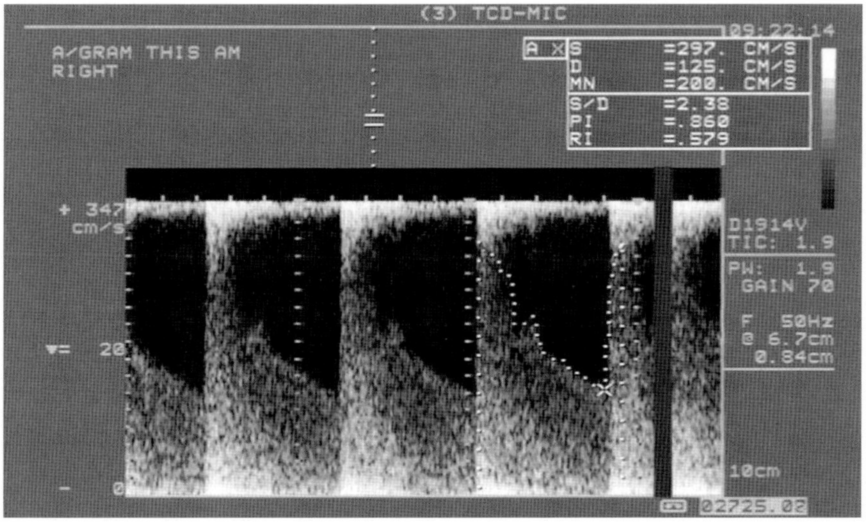

FIGURE 10.2. Transcranial Doppler. Doppler spectrum shows double shape as a result of mirror image artifact.

Artifact: Mirror image artifact of Doppler spectrum. A mirror image of a Doppler spectrum can appear on the opposite side of the baseline when the flow is unidirectional and should appear on only one side of the baseline. This is an electronic duplication of the spectral information, and it can occur when receiver gain is set too high or when the Doppler angle is near 90 degrees. This occurs because beams are focused and not cylindrical in shape, such that portions of the beam can experience approaching flow and other parts can experience receding flow (2).

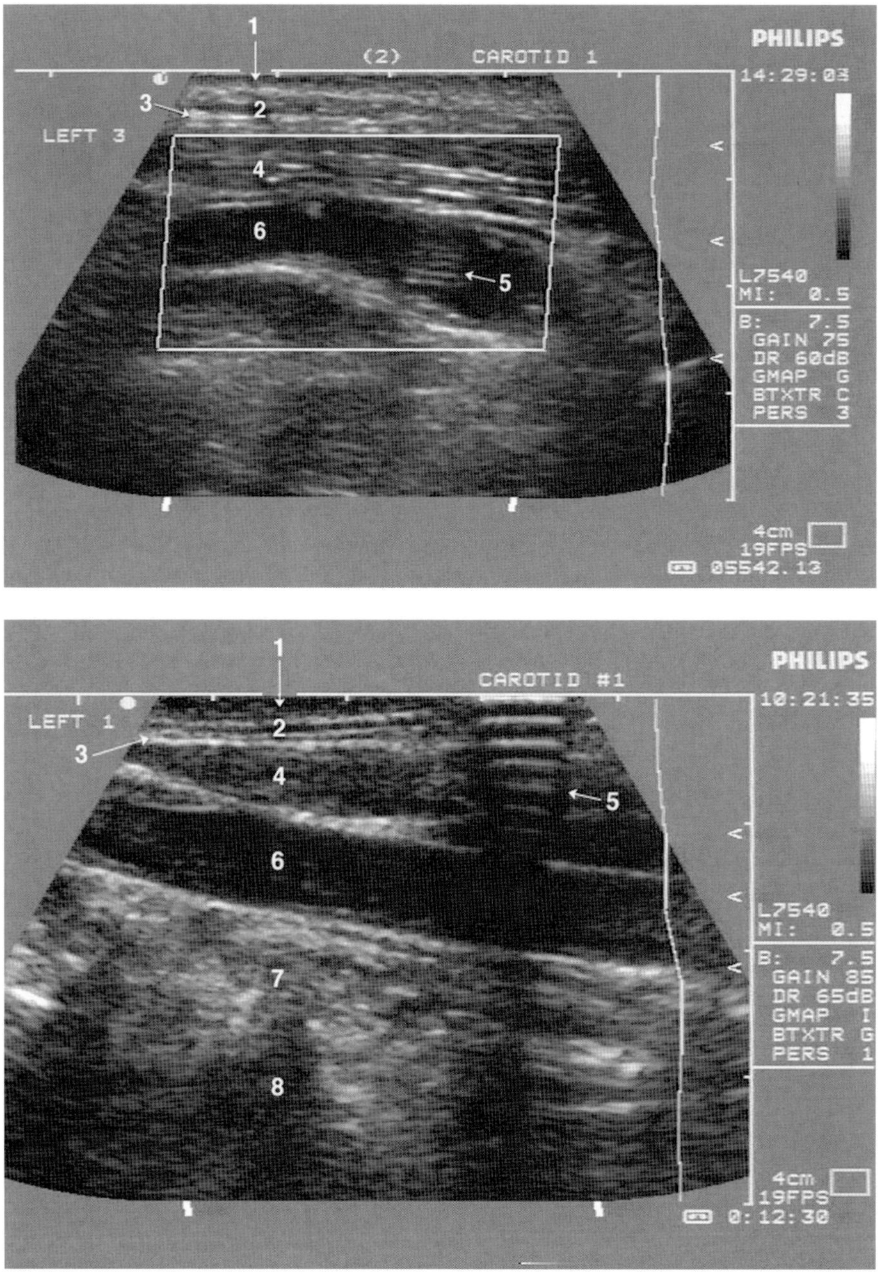

FIGURE 10.3. A: Left common carotid artery. Posterolateral view. Longitudinal. Gray scale. *1*, Skin and superficial cervical fascia; *2*, platysma; *3*, deep cervical fascia; *4*, sternocleidomastoid muscle; *5*, reverberation (artifact); *6*, left common carotid artery. **B:** Left common carotid artery. Anteroposterior view. Longitudinal. Gray scale. *1*, Skin and superficial cervical fascia; *2*, platysma; *3*, deep cervical fascia; *4*, sternocleidomastoid muscle; *5*, reverberation (artifact); *6*, left common carotid artery; *7*, longus colli and scalenus anterior muscles; *8*, shadow.

Artifact: Reverberation. If two or more reflectors are encountered in the sound path, multiple reflections occur. The echoes represent subsequent echoes from traversing the path between two reflectors several times. They are placed behind the second real reflector at separation intervals equal to the separation between the first and second real reflectors. Each subsequent reflection is weaker than prior ones. The first of the two reflectors is usually the transducer face (3).

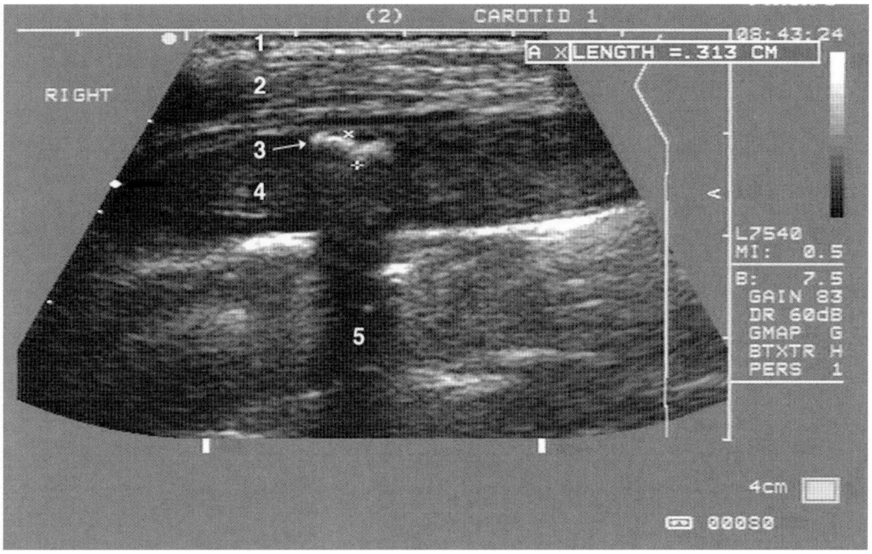

FIGURE 10.4. Bifurcation of the right common carotid artery. Lateral view. Longitudinal. Gray scale. *1,* Skin and superficial cervical fascia; *2,* sternocleidomastoid muscle; *3,* calcific plaque in the near wall of the bifurcation of the right common carotid artery; *4,* right common carotid artery; *5,* shadowing.

Artifact: Shadowing. Shadowing is the reduced amplitude of echoes caused by intervening structures with high attenuation. A pronounced shadow distal to a calcific plaque is shown in the figure. The plaque is very echogenic, indicating a strong reflection. This, in addition to the larger absorption in the calcific plaque, causes weak echoes of tissues distally (4).

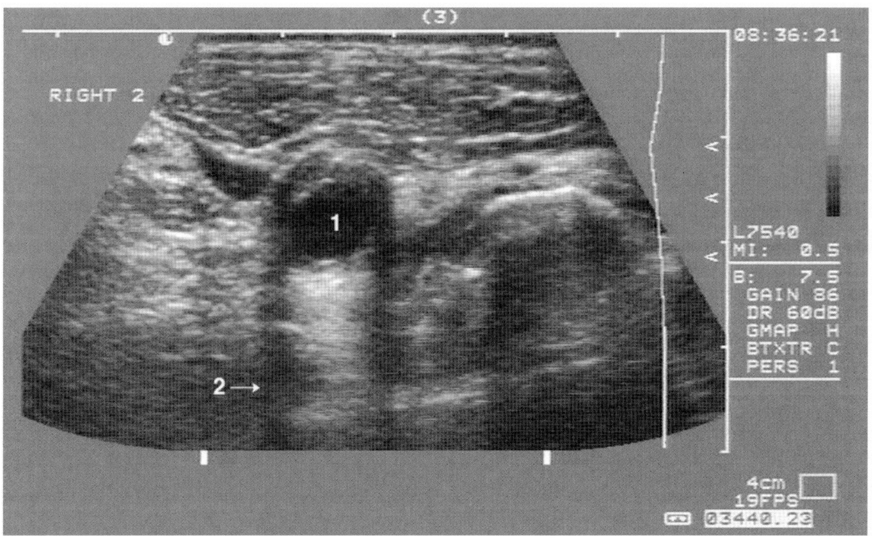

FIGURE 10.5. Right common carotid artery. Transverse view. Gray scale. *1,* Right common carotid artery; *2,* refraction (edge) shadowing.

Artifact: Refraction (edge) shadowing. Shadowing from the edge of a curved object can occur as a result of refraction, which is not necessarily a strong or weak attenuators. The cause may be the defocusing action of a refracting curved surface, and the shadow results from reduced intensity as the beam spreads after refraction (5).

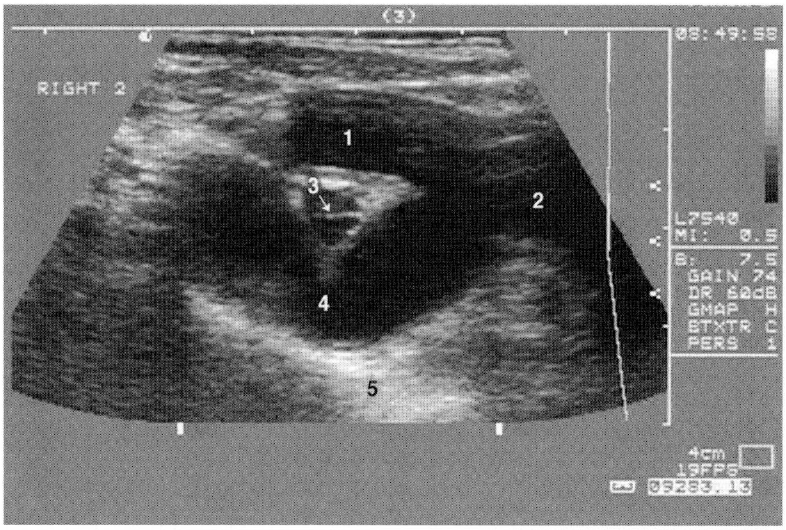

FIGURE 10.6. Right internal jugular vein and brachiocephalic artery. Transverse view. Gray scale. *1*, Right common carotid artery; *2*, innominate artery; *3*, right internal jugular vein and jugular valve; *4*, right subclavian artery; *5*, enhancement.

Diagnosis: Artifacts in ultrasound imaging. Enhancement. Enhancement is the increased relative amplitude of echoes from reflectors that lie behind weakly attenuating structures. Enhancement from the low attenuation of blood in the common carotid, jugular vein, and subclavian artery is seen in the figure (3).

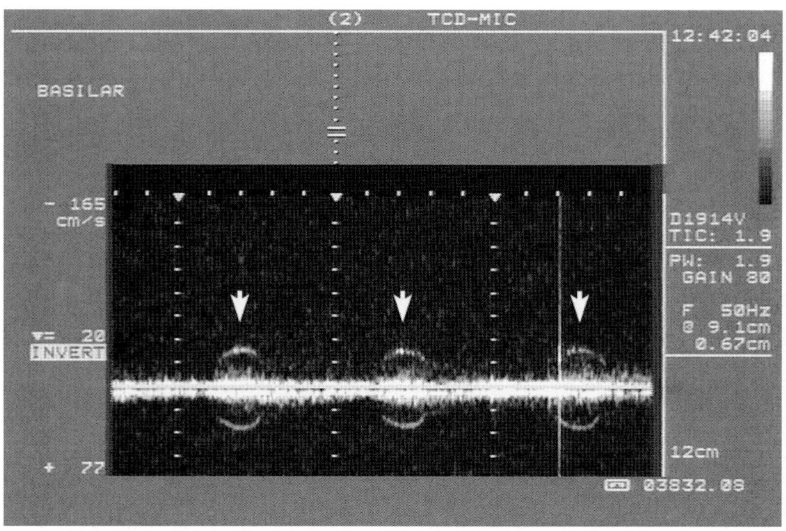

FIGURE 10.7. Transcranial Doppler sonography. Doppler spectrum at the level of the basilar artery showing the wall motion (*arrowheads*).

Diagnosis: Artifacts caused by improper equipment settings. Some artifacts are produced by improper equipment operation or settings. To eliminate the high-intensity, low-frequency Doppler shift echoes (clutter) resulting from the motion of the vessel wall, a high-pass wall filter is used. When this filter setting is lower than the low-frequency Doppler shift echoes, the artifacts appear in the image (1).

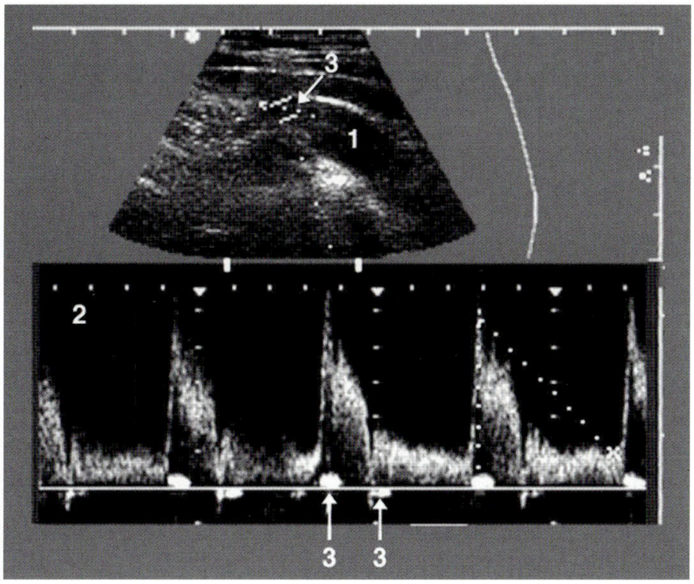

FIGURE 10.8. Right brachiocephalic artery. Lateral view. Longitudinal. Gray scale. Doppler spectrum. *1,* Sample placed at the right brachiocephalic artery; *2,* Doppler spectrum of the brachiocephalic artery; *3,* wall motion artifact.

Diagnosis: Wall motion artifact. The high-intensity, low-frequency Doppler shift echoes resulting from heart or vessel wall and cardiac valve motion with pulsatile flow are called *clutter.* In vascular studies, a high-pass wall filter or wall-thump filter rejects the frequencies below an adjustable value, thus eliminating the clutter. These strong echoes have low Doppler shift frequencies because the walls of the brachiocephalic artery do not move as fast as the blood does. The wall-thump filter should be used with caution because it can alter the data regarding diastolic flow (2).

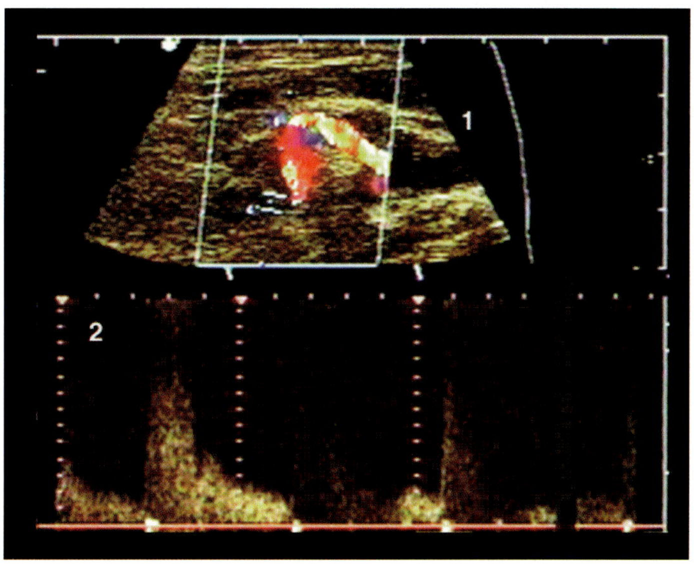

FIGURE 10.9. Left internal carotid artery. Lateral view. Longitudinal. B-color scale. Doppler spectrum. *1,* Sample volume placed at the left internal carotid artery; *2,* Doppler spectrum of the left internal carotid artery.

Diagnosis: Contrast resolution versus color artifact. Some instruments have the ability to present different echo intensities in various colors. Because the eye can differentiate more color tints than gray shades, color displays offer improved contrast resolution capability. In this case, the color was assigned dark orange through yellow to white. This process is called *B-color* or *B-color scale* (6).

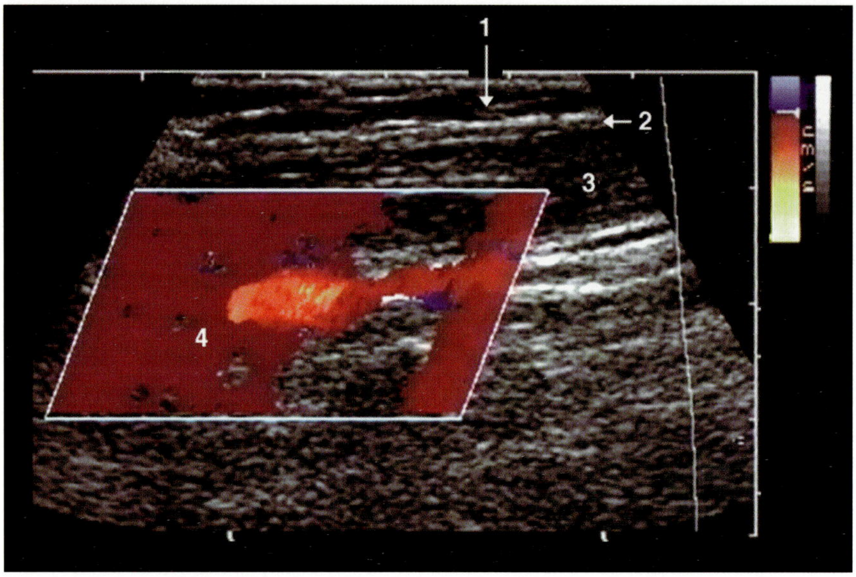

FIGURE 10.10. Right internal carotid artery. Lateral view. Longitudinal. Color. *1*, Skin and superficial cervical fascia; *2*, platysma and deep cervical fascia; *3*, sternocleidomastoid muscle; *4*, color artifact.

Diagnosis: Color movement artifact. With color duplex imaging, anything within the field-of-view that moves relative to the transducer is represented in color. This phenomenon is known as color flash, and the problem is caused by the movement of the transducer by the operator (7).

PEARLS AND PITFALLS

Pearls

- Aliasing is the most common artifact encountered in Doppler ultrasound and it indicates the improper representation of Doppler shift information that has been insufficiently sampled.
- Some ultrasound imaging artifacts are useful in interpretation and diagnosis, whereas some can cause confusion and error.
- Shadowing and enhancement are two useful artifacts that belong to the attenuation group. They assist in determining the cystic nature of echogenic fluid collections.
- Ultrasound imaging artifacts of acoustic origin can be classified based on the inherent nature of the ultrasound.

Pitfalls

- The mirror image artifact of Doppler spectrum is an electronic duplication of the spectral information that occurs when receiver gain is set too high. It can lead to misinterpretation of the measurement of flow parameters.
- Because ultrasound beams are focused and not cylindrical in shape, portions of the beam can experience flow toward while other portions can experience flow away when the straight vessel is scanned by a perpendicular beam. This affects the color display despite a constant direction and velocity of flow.
- To eliminate high-intensity, low-frequency Doppler shift echoes resulting from heart or vessel wall motion, a high-pass wall filter or wall-thump filter is used. It should be used with caution to avoid misinterpreting diastolic flow.
- A more important source of error relating to improper equipment setting artifacts is the nonvisualization of slow poststenotic flow, which occurs when the high-pass wall filter is set lower than the low-frequency Doppler shift echoes.

QUESTIONS

1. Aliasing
   a. is the most common artifact encountered in Doppler ultrasound.
   b. indicates the improper representation of Doppler shift information that has been insufficiently sampled.
   c. occurs when the true Doppler shift exceeds one half of the pulse repetition frequency.
   d. All of the above
   e. None of the above

2. The mirror image artifact of Doppler spectrum is an electronic duplication of the spectral information and can occur when the receiver gain is set too high or when the Doppler angle is near 90 degrees.
   True or false?

3. Reverberation is an artifact in ultrasound imaging in which
   a. multiple refractions occur because two or more reflectors are encountered in the sound path.
   b. each subsequent reflection is weaker than prior ones.
   c. the first of the two refractors is usually the transducer face.
   d. All of the above
   e. None of the above

4. Shadowing is the reduced amplitude of echoes caused by intervening structures with low attenuation.
   True or false?

5. Edge shadowing is an artifact caused by
   a. strong attenuators.
   b. strong reflectors.
   c. strong refractors.
   d. All of the above
   e. None of the above

6. Enhancement is the increased relative amplitude of echoes from reflectors that lie behind weakly attenuating structures.
   True or false?

7. Improper equipment setting artifacts occur when the high-pass wall filter is set ________ than the ________ frequency Doppler shift echoes.
   a. lower, high-
   b. lower, low-
   c. higher, low-
   d. higher, high-
   e. None of the above

8. The left common carotid artery (Fig. 10.11) appears to have no flow (no color within it) at the level of its bifurcation. This occurs because
   a. there is a calcific plaque in the near wall of the bifurcation.
   b. low echogenicity material filling the left bifurcation produces an occlusion of the vessel lumen.
   c. the Doppler angle between the flow and the scan lines at that point is close to 90 degrees and color flow is often not detected in that situation.

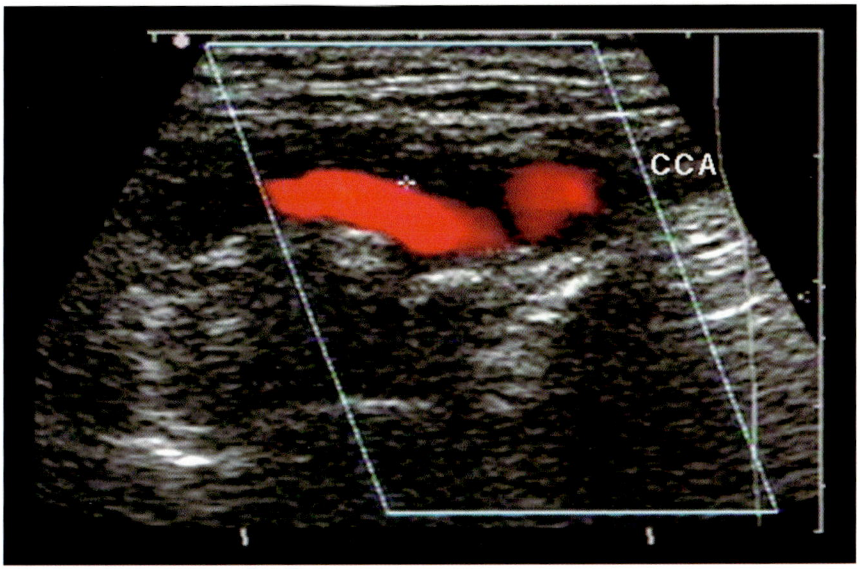

FIGURE 10.11. Bifurcation of the left common carotid artery (CCA). Lateral view. Longitudinal. Color.

d. All of the above
e. None of the above

9. Match the name with the number of the artifact that appears in Figure 10.12.
   a. Edge shadowing
   b. Refraction shadowing
   c. Enhancement

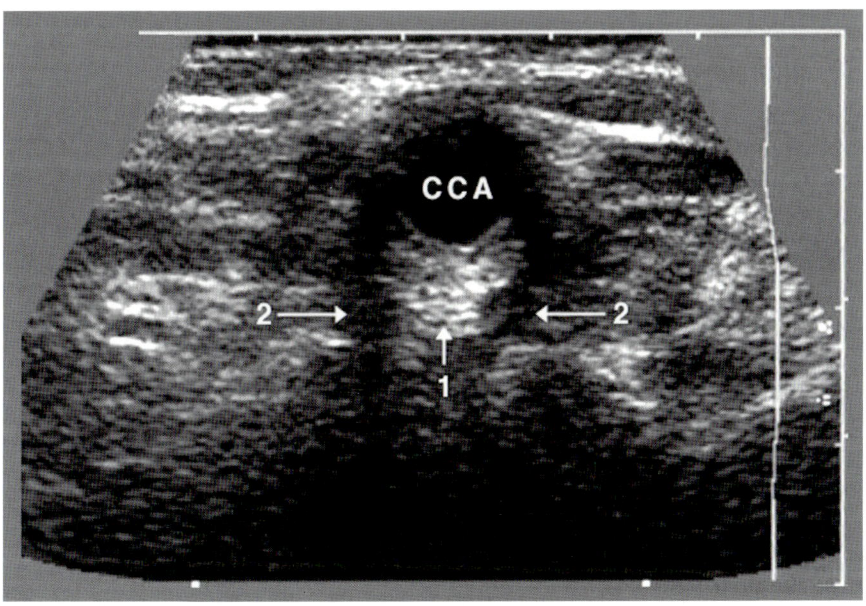

FIGURE 10.12. Right common carotid artery. Transverse view. Gray scale.

Answers: **1.** d; **2.** True; **3.** b; **4.** False; **5.** c; **6.** True; **7.** b; **8.** c; **9.** a.

REFERENCES

1. Kremkau FW. *Diagnostic ultrasound. Principles and instruments,* 4th ed. Philadelphia: WB Saunders, 1993.
2. Kremkau FW. *Diagnostic ultrasound. Principles and instruments,* 5th ed. Philadelphia: WB Saunders, 1998.
3. Kremkau FW, Taylor KJW. Artifacts in ultrasound imaging. *J Ultrasound Med* 1986;5: 227–237.
4. Mitchell SE, Gross BH, Spitz HB. The hypoechoic caudate lobe: an ultrasonic pseudolesion. *Radiology* 1982;144:569.
5. Sommer FG, Filly RA, Minton MJ. Acoustic shadowing due to refractive and reflective effects. *Am J Roentgenol* 1979;132:973.
6. Pizer SM, Zimmerman JB. Color display in ultrasonography. *Ultrasound Med Biol* 1983;9:331–345.
7. Zwiebel WJ. Color-encoded blood flow imaging. *Semin Ultrasound CT MR* 1988;9: 324.

SUBJECT INDEX

Note: Page numbers followed by F indicate figures: page numbers followed by t indicate tables.